Person-Centered Planning Made Easy

Person-Centered Planning Made Easy
The PICTURE Method

by

Steve Holburn, Ph.D.

New York State Institute for Basic Research in Developmental Disabilities
Staten Island

Anne Gordon, M.S.Ed.

New York State Institute for Basic Research in Developmental Disabilities
Staten Island

and

Peter M. Vietze, Ph.D.

Hand In Hand Development
New York
John F. Kennedy Jr. Institute for Worker Education
City University of New York

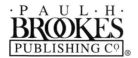

·P·A·U·L·H·
BROOKES
PUBLISHING Co.®

Baltimore • London • Sydney

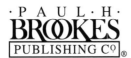

Paul H. Brookes Publishing Co.
Post Office Box 10624
Baltimore, Maryland 21285-0624

www.brookespublishing.com

Typeset by Auburn Associates, Inc., Baltimore, Maryland.
Manufactured in the United States of America by
Integrated Books International, Dulles, Virginia.

The individuals described in this book are composites or real people whose
situations have been masked and are based on the authors' experiences.
Names and identifying details have been changed to protect confidentiality.

The photographs that appear on the cover and throughout the book are used
by permission of the individuals pictured or their parents or guardians.

Second printing, November, 2016.

Library of Congress Cataloging-in-Publication Data
Holburn, Steve.
  Person-centered planning made easy: the PICTURE method / by
Charles Steven Holburn, Anne Gordon, Peter M. Vietze.
     p.   cm.
  Includes bibliographical references and index.
  ISBN-13: 978-1-55766-853-0
  ISBN-10: 1-55766-853-1
  1. People with disabilities—Services for.   2. Sociology of disability.
  I. Gordon, Anne.   II. Vietze, Peter, 1944–.   III. Title.
  HV1568.H65 2006
  362.4'048—dc22

                                              2006027845

British Library Cataloguing in Publication data are available from the British
Library.

Contents

Step 3: Plan a Better Future

Step 4: Implement the Plan

Person-Centered Organizational Capacity Indicators: Increasing Organizational
Capacity for Person-Centered Outcomes

About the Authors

Steve Holburn, Ph.D., BCBA, Head, Intervention Research Laboratory, New York State Institute for Basic Research in Developmental Disabilities, 1050 Forest Hill Road, Staten Island, NY, 10314

Steve Holburn is Head of the Intervention Research Laboratory at the New York State Institute for Basic Research in Developmental Disabilities and is also a Board Certified Behavior Analyst at Association for the Help of Retarded Children in New York City. He has written extensively in the field of developmental disabilities services, including areas such as person-centered planning, residential regulations, quality of life, health promotion, self-injurious behavior, assistive technology, and parents with intellectual disabilities. A priority research aim of the Intervention Research Laboratory has been the discovery of person-centered planning approaches that can be effectively implemented within existing developmental service systems. Accordingly, Dr. Holburn has used the methods of applied behavior analysis and program evaluation, often in combination, in conducting research towards this end. The blending of person-centered planning with traditional professional practice has yielded procedures foundational to the PICTURE method of person-centered planning.

Dr. Holburn's work in person-centered planning has garnered international interest, and many of his publications have been translated into various languages. Examples of international influence include assisting in the planning of deinstitutionalization now underway in Japan, evaluating service efficiency for the Hong Kong government, and helping the Thailand Department of Mental Health to adopt person-centered principles and methods.

Anne Gordon, M.S.Ed., Educator and Researcher, New York State Institute for Basic Research in Developmental Disabilities, 1050 Forest Hill Road, Staten Island, NY, 10314

Anne Gordon is an educator and researcher at the New York State Institute for Basic Research in Developmental Disabilities. She began her career as Director of the Early Childhood Direction Center of Staten Island and then moved on to become Director of the Staten Island Early Intervention Service Coordination Office. In those capacities, she assisted parents of children with developmental disabilities to connect to, and advocate for, early intervention and preschool special education services. She has conducted person-centered planning evaluation research on implementing person-centered planning with parents who have developmental disabilities, and young adults with autism, transitioning from high school to the adult world. In addition, Ms. Gordon conducts person-centered planning workshops to local and international audiences, focusing on implementing the approach within their existing structures. Ms. Gordon is a co-author of the *Health Advocacy Program: An Activity-Based Curriculum for Adults with Developmental Disabilities* and is the facilitator of the Staten Island Down Syndrome Parent Support Group. She is also the parent of a young adult with Down syndrome.

Peter M. Vietze, Ph.D., Director of Research and Development, Hand In Hand Development, 465 Grand Street, Second Floor, New York, NY 10002; Senior Research Associate, John F. Kennedy Jr. Institute for Worker Education, City University of New York, 101 West 31st Street, 14th Floor, New York, NY 10001

Peter M. Vietze is currently Director of Research and Development at Hand In Hand Development, an early intervention agency, and Senior Research Associate at the John F. Kennedy Jr. Institute for Worker Education. Dr. Vietze is also Executive Director of Community Assistance Resources and Extended Services, a not-for-profit community agency serving New York's Lower East Side and Washington Heights. He received his doctorate in 1969 from Wayne State University, where he concentrated on developmental psychology and social psychology. After a postdoctoral year at University of California, Berkeley, conducting research on infant behavior, he landed a faculty position at George Peabody College, where he directed Head Start research with parents, conducted research with infants, young children, and their parents and directed the Developmental Psychology training program. Dr. Vietze worked at the National Institutes of Health for 11 years as a research scientist and also as Head of the Mental Retardation Research Centers Program. From 1987 to 2004, Dr. Vietze was Executive Deputy Director and the 1st Chair of the Department of Infant Development of the New York State Institute for Basic Research in Developmental Disabilities (IBR). During the last 10 years of his tenure at IBR, Dr. Vietze collaborated with Dr. Holburn and Ms. Gordon on several person-centered planning projects, including the Willowbrook Futures Project and the Parent Resource Project. Most recently, Dr. Vietze and Ms.Gordon applied their knowledge of person-centered planning to a group of 33 transition-age youngsters and their families. Dr. Vietze has published more than 100 chapters and journal articles in a variety of topics in early development, developmental disabilities, and child abuse. The New York State Department of Health recently released evidence-based clinical practice guidelines for infants and toddlers with Down syndrome developed by a panel of experts that Dr. Vietze chaired.

Foreword

Developmental disabilities first emerged as an organized field out of a commitment to support individuals with physical and intellectual disabilities who have difficulty communicating, learning, working and building the social relationships that are critical to a rich quality of life. With this book, Holburn, Gordon, and Vietze offer a step-by-step approach for organizing support using a person-centered vision. There are several elements of this practical handbook that are worthy of note.

The first and most important element is the focus on organizing support for an individual around the quality of life vision of the person, not around diagnostic or professional criteria. Early efforts to provide support for people with developmental disabilities emphasized what was possible. Research demonstrated that people with disabilities (even those with severe disabilities) were able to learn, perform, and benefit from education and support far beyond what was initially assumed. Rather than futures of sheltered care, a future of rich relationships, work, leisure, learning, and play were both possible and expected. Recognizing the abilities of people with disabilities has been an enormous challenge for the field. Instead of organizing systems of support around professional opinion and diagnostic criteria, we are now faced with the wonderful challenge of organizing support around the preferences, competencies, and personal visions of those who receive support. This transformation from a professional-centered to a person-centered approach to support is still in process. There are ongoing debates about the value of professionally delivered supports, and the hindrance that is possible even if advocates (e.g., family) guide support rather than the person him/herself. What this book makes clear is that individual supports 1) make a difference and should be valued, organized, and recruited, 2) will be most efficient and effective if they are organized and guided by a clear vision of the personal competence, preference, and vision of the individual receiving support, and 3) may be delivered by both professional and informal sources using practices that are evidence based. The fundamental message is that support should be person centered in both form and function.

The second major contribution of the book is to reassert the importance of overall quality of life as the foundation for support. Early efforts to assist individuals with disabilities overemphasized the development of skills and abilities without ensuring that these gains transformed into functional lifestyle outcomes. It is wonderful to be able to dress yourself but much better if you have the chance to use that skill on a regular basis and you actually enjoy the clothes you put on. The pioneers in person-centered planning offered a radical and obvious message: The value of support lies in the impact it has on the quality of a person's life. The problem that message created is that while few would argue with the vision, it was not clear how to assess quality of life, or a person's preferences for quality of life. Holburn et al. offer credible (and still developing) strategies for not just assessing quality of life once, but also for repeated reassessment and adjustment. We have all experienced the curse of getting exactly what we asked for and realizing it was not what we expected. Life is about turns and twists, not straight lines. As a result, support needs to adjust and adapt to meet these turns and twists.

Holburn et al. challenge us with a vision in which person-centered planning is not an event that occurs at one point in time, but is a repeated process that commands continued alterations as a person's life emerges. The altering focus and forms that support takes are tied consistently to the personal vision of the individual. That vision will not always lead in directions that parents, family, advocates, or professionals would choose, but also it leads to a more rich and personal life.

A third feature of this book is the commitment to research-based practices. This is a challenging perspective for a book focused on person-centered planning. The conceptual and theoretical foundation for person-centered planning far outstrips the hard evidence for effectiveness. As readers, we are fortunate in that these authors have provided among the most rigorous assessments of person-centered planning and the effects of this approach on the features of support and impact on quality of life. There remains, however, a great deal to be done before person-centered planning can be touted as an evidence-based practice. It is a logical approach with strong evaluation outcomes. The very focus on large impact, however, makes the approach a challenge to study using conventional research methods. Holburn et al. provide an elegant balance in their description of what is known and what is recommended. By providing clear, specific descriptions of the steps that should be followed in person-centered planning, they make a major contribution to those who accept that task of systematically assessing the impact of these procedures.

The PICTURE approach to person-centered planning offers one model among many person-centered tools available today. PICTURE blends professional and informal supports and requires iterative strategies for modifying support plans. These are useful features to emphasize, but the major contribution of this book is to provide a detailed, operational description of how to deliver person-centered planning. This book is not likely to be sufficient for someone without training to conduct person-centered planning—there simply is too much background. But the book will be of tremendous value for those who have mastered the main ideas and are looking for the organizational practices that bring those ideas to life. In the end, we all wish that the practices and vision of this book will result in people with disabilities leading lives that are more rich, complete, and consistent with their personal preferences.

Robert Horner, Ph.D.
Alumni-Knight Professor
Special Education, College of Education
University of Oregon

Preface

Person-centered planning has become a movement in the field of developmental disabilities, and many agencies that serve people with disabilities are trying to adopt it as their general approach to service provision. Few can argue with the principles and goals of person-centered planning, yet with the myriad approaches available and the dearth of empirical research on person-centered planning, it is difficult for an agency administrator to know which approaches work best and how they can be applied most realistically in an agency. We think this is because person-centered planning has not undergone an evolution typical of other interventions whose methods are subject to change on the basis of trial and error. However, we have not been afraid to experiment with our own variations, the result of which has culminated in this book, *Person-Centered Planning Made Easy: The PICTURE Method,* which represents the best of what we have learned in 15 years of implementing and evaluating person-centered planning.

We developed PICTURE to be practical and effective for developmental services agencies. It is a system-friendly approach that provides feedback to keep the process moving forward. PICTURE does not try to supplant an agency's current mission and procedures for helping people have high-quality lives—it blends with existing agency processes, and it can make them more efficient and effective. The book provides straightforward instructions and illustrations, as it guides the team, step-by-step, in shifting more power to the person.

When I was first introduced to person-centered planning, I knew this was something big. The principles were fresh and simple. I was struck by the enthusiasm of the facilitator and the clarity of the vision that she crafted with a cooperative yet somewhat skeptical team. I was an observer. The vision was for William to leave the institution so that he could live with his sister, and the team was discussing a house addition suited to his preferences. I questioned whether this could actually happen. William had a reputation for hurting people, and he spent parts of his day being guarded by staff. Nonetheless, the planning plowed forward, despite a few disengaged clinicians, whose involvement did not seem necessary at the time. Then William had two unsuccessful home visits that frightened his sister, and his behavior took a turn for the worse. Eventually the process fizzled out, and William never did move in with his sister. A few months later, a member of the defunct person-centered planning team told me about some significant positive changes in William's life that resulted from the process, and he wanted to know why the person-centered planning had stopped.

I pondered this planning failure. First, it appeared that critical professionals were overlooked. In retrospect, William did not have enough technical support to succeed. Would the home visits at his sister's house have succeeded if a behavior analyst had accompanied William? Second, it was clear that the team had not been cohesive enough to survive adversity. Would more problem solving or better knowledge of the team's own positive results have kept the process alive? My observations about William's short-lived person-centered planning planted the seeds of PICTURE's development.

We have had a long time to improve upon the person-centered planning process. Ill-fated processes, like the just mentioned, have taught my colleagues and me a great deal about what doesn't work in person-centered planning. More importantly, we have used these failures as opportunities for improvement, and we have experimented with new ways to affect enhancements to quality of life. This book represents a collection of methods, that together, constitute the evolution of our own variations that have proven most effective. We hope that users of this book will continue this process of change by devising further improvements and sharing them with others.

A note about terminology is in order here. We have used the words *person* and *individual* throughout the manual in referring to the person with a disability. Occasionally, to distinguish between staff members and the person with the disability, we have used more conventional terminology, such as *person with a disability* or referents containing the terms *developmental disability* and *intellectual disability*.

Acknowledgments

Many of the concepts and procedures described in this manual were directly influenced by the originators of person-centered planning. In particular, John O'Brien, Connie Lyle O'Brien, and Beth Mount have had the greatest influence on our thinking. They have been true leaders in the recent changing landscape of developmental services. We also wish to acknowledge other individuals who influenced the development of PICTURE, and who have had a significant impact on person-centered organizational change throughout the United States. These individuals include Allen Schwartz, Don Kincaid, Dennis Reid, Al Pfadt, John Jacobson, and Bernard Carabello. We also wish to thank our international friends who piloted prototype versions of this manual in introducing person-centered planning in their own countries. Here, special thanks go to Noriaki Tekeda and Ryosei Ohya from Japan and Suchada Sakornsatian and Nantana Ratanakorn from Thailand.

Particular tribute goes to Sal and Ida Giordano and their son Sal. Their devotion to getting things right served as an inspiration to many people in the downstate New York area interested in developing individualized services for people with disabilities. Finally, we extend a special thanks to Christian Gordon, who has shared his life with us during his own person-centered planning, some of which appears as examples and photographs in the manual.

To the parents with intellectual disabilities and their children who helped us understand the importance of professional support and evaluation in making person-centered planning work. Thank you, Lana, Nina, Tom, Brenda, Linda, and Sakinah.

Person-Centered Planning Made Easy

PART I

Person-Centered Planning and PICTURE

This manual describes how to implement person-centered planning and is intended to help people with disabilities achieve more satisfying lifestyles. The *Planning for Inclusive Communities Together Using Reinforcement and Evaluation* (PICTURE) approach was designed for people who are receiving services from human services agencies; thus, the manual is a guide for agencies that want to systematically implement person-centered planning. In a nutshell, in using the PICTURE method of person-centered planning, a handful of people who care about a person ask three main questions: "What is your life like now?" "How do you want it to change?" and "How can we help make that happen?"

There are other manuals on person-centered planning, but this one is different. In our 10 years of conducting, teaching, and researching this method, we have departed from some of the original tenets of the process in reaching for better outcomes for greater numbers of people. In doing so, we discovered some things that have been helpful, and we have incorporated these variations into our own person-centered planning techniques, which we have assembled in this manual.

We hope that you find this method an efficient and effective way to help a person make significant life changes. Specifically, PICTURE incorporates much of the existing professional thought and practice in the field of intellectual disabilities, including interventions such as teaching techniques, therapeutic procedures, and applied behavior analysis. The steps of the PICTURE process are defined, and a method for assessing adherence to that process is given. Perhaps most important, we provide objective measurement tools that inform both the person-centered team and the agency management team of the outcomes of their planning. This feedback is used to make adjustments in management response and team planning. We have introduced a few scientific principles into person-centered planning and have retained the essential person-centered planning practices that were described in the early development of the process during the 1980s. In departing from some of the original precepts (see Mount & Patterson, 1986; O'Brien, 1987; O'Brien & O'Brien, 2002; Yates, 1980), we acknowledge that we are contributing to a process that was pioneered by others. However, this poses no problem because our goal is not better person-centered planning per se; it is better lives for people with disabilities. By better lives we mean more autonomy, better relationships, a more pleasant living environment, and a true social contribution. We believe that if you follow the steps in this manual, you are likely to significantly improve the quality of living for people with disabilities. An agency that facilitates this process will inevitably discover methods of deploying professional and support staff in ways that are more satisfying to people with disabilities, workers, and family members.

A BRIEF HISTORY OF PERSON-CENTERED PLANNING: WHAT IS PERSON-CENTERED PLANNING AND WHERE DID IT COME FROM?

Person-centered planning is a way of helping undervalued people, such as people with intellectual disabilities, get what they need and want in their lives. Because such people are often segregated from the rest of us, person-centered planning emphasizes social inclusion of people with disabilities, which has become a movement in many Western cultures. In fact, the ideological foundations of person-centered planning can be found in the principles of normalization (Nirje, 1969; Wolfensberger, 1972), which were presented at least a decade before the person-centered planning approach was developed. However, person-centered planning offers something more than a theoretical framework and good ideas. It prescribes a way to turn the ideologies of normalization and social inclusion into realities. Thus, person-centered planning blends together an ideology about the types of changes that *should* occur with a strategy on *how* to bring about those changes.

Person-centered planning emerged in the mid-1990s as a way to better understand the experiences of people with developmental disabilities and, with the help of others, to expand and enhance those experiences (O'Brien & Lovett, 1992; O'Brien, O'Brien, & Mount, 1997). More specifically, person-centered planning attempts to reduce social isolation, foster friendships, increase opportunities for preferred activities, develop competence, and promote respect. Policy makers and service agencies in the United States, Canada, and the United Kingdom have embraced its tenets with vigor (Holburn & Vietze, 1999; Schwartz, Jacobson, & Holburn, 2000), but the actual process of carrying out person-centered planning as described by its founders is neither brief nor easy, and, consequently, person-centered planning is often misapplied in service systems that have tried to adopt it (O'Brien et al., 1997).

GOALS OF PERSON-CENTERED PLANNING

The goals of person-centered planning most commonly referred to are the five essential accomplishments described by O'Brien (1987) and are defined briefly here.

1. Community presence: Being in an ordinary place, such as a typical neighborhood or an integrated classroom

2. Community participation: Being among the person's network of community friends and allies

3. Choice: Having autonomy in making decisions about everyday matters

4. Respect: Having a valued role in community life

5. Competence: Being able to do the things that contribute to respect

These are laudable goals for people with intellectual disabilities, and appear to have universal appeal in the disabilities field. However, there are two limitations to this set of goals. First, these goals were not developed by the people for whom they are intended; they are offered by others who are speaking for people with disabilities. Second, because person-centered planning grew out of concerns about the problems of institutional living for people with developmental disabilities, the goals reflect the deprivations experienced by people who were confined or incarcerated. Therefore, these goals might not be completely consistent with those of the person whom you might be assisting. Nonetheless, in our planning, we rarely encounter individuals whose aspirations do not fit into some of these areas. The point here is that we need to listen closely to the desires of the person we are trying to help, regardless of our preconceptions about what would make for a better quality of life for that person.

A SNAPSHOT OF THE PERSON-CENTERED PLANNING PROCESS

Person-centered planning is a multifaceted, long-term intervention that requires a large amount of problem solving and organizational accommodation. Basically, person-centered planning brings together the most important people in the life of a person, envisions a better life for the person, and discovers ways to achieve the vision. The team should have a diverse composition and should not consist solely of human service workers. The team should not resemble the traditional interdisciplinary clinical team planning process in which professional authority prevails to ameliorate or eliminate the person's deficiencies. Instead, the views of the person with a disability, family members, and friends should be paramount, and the planning is less of a corrective undertaking than an attempt to establish a better life for the person. Much, but not all, of the decision making shifts from the service system employees to the person with the disability. In person-centered planning, power and decision making are shared.

What kind of plan is produced when the planning process is driven by the person with a disability? It does not look like a typical interdisciplinary program because the plan content is neither mandated by a higher authority, nor do the goals reflect a set of

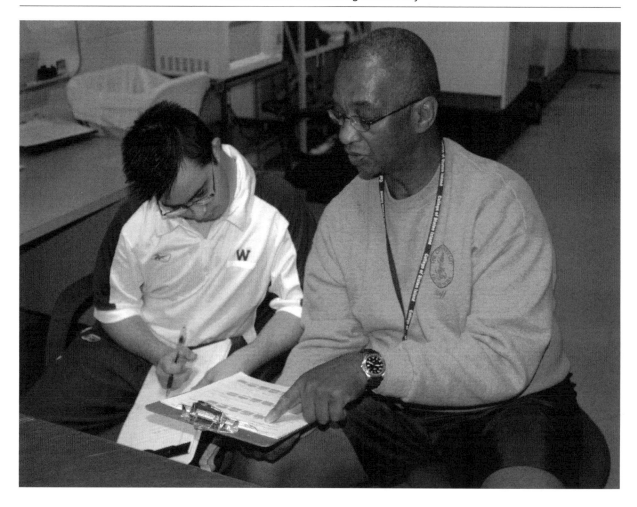

predetermined health and skill areas that need to be assessed and addressed. In traditional systems, plans and services for people with developmental disabilities are often
ineffective because the planning must accommodate regulations that are often arbitrary
and fixed service patterns that are governed by funding sources, clinical convention,
and even the convenience of the service providers. In person-centered planning, the
planning is governed by the person with a disability, who is at the center of the planning process. All other considerations must be made secondary. Nonetheless, the plan
must contain conventional elements such as realistic objectives, strategies for carrying
out the plan, and accountability. An effective plan includes clear steps and requirements
that lead to the realization of the person's vision or dream.

As one might expect, a great deal of group problem solving takes place in person-
centered planning because although the person's aspirations might not correspond to
the services offered by the service organization, he or she still needs the support of the
organization. Thus, another step in person-centered planning occurs when the team
confronts the obstacle in which the organization does not provide what the person
wants in its existing program. Therefore, the person-centered team must problem-solve
and devise ways of making the person's dream become a reality. The team does not do
this independently; it encourages the organization to support the dream. Organizational
change within the service agency may be necessary, especially if multiple person-
centered planning endeavors are taking place within the agency. Person-centered plan-

ning will expand in an agency if the organization is able to accommodate this new way of helping.

The problem solving necessary to help the person achieve a better life is guided by a facilitator, who runs planning meetings and keeps the group focused on core goals and values, such as inclusion, friendships, and personal autonomy. The facilitator often records or charts what people say on large sheets of paper. The information is organized by themes that capture the person's experiences, interests, dreams, and so forth; and this information becomes the basis for developing a plan for a better future. Through consensus, the facilitator identifies ways to accomplish the plan and secures commitments for follow-through.

The group meets periodically to reflect on successes and setbacks and to make adjustments in strategy. There are no set rules for how often the team should meet or how long person-centered planning should last. This is up to the team and the person. It is important for the group to remain intact until the major goals are achieved. After that, team members might meet periodically to find out how the person is doing and to offer their continued support where needed.

BUREAUCRATIC SYSTEMS AND PERSON-CENTERED PLANNING

Bureaucracies are typically viewed as organizations run by formal processes, standardization, and multiple hierarchical approval procedures. Such systems bring to mind inefficiency and waste. A bureaucracy is sometimes said to exist solely for itself and to achieve results that end up in enlarging the size of the bureaucracy. In the developmental services area, bureaucratic systems have developed practices that maintain the person as a *client* in a protected but relatively isolated lifestyle, and changes to the contrary require approvals from many levels and divisions of management. Such procedural safeguards have the effect of discouraging the innovation needed to bring about improvements in a person's quality of life. Alternatively, the person-centered approach encourages social inclusion of a *citizen* with a less supervised lifestyle. In doing so, it deliberately promotes organization changes that accommodate a person's aspirations. The contrasts in Table 1 illustrate the differences in the goals and planning practices of these two organizing frameworks. Note that the person-centered approach appears more fundamental and certainly less technical,

Table 1. Bureaucratic systems versus person-centered systems

Bureaucratic system	Person-centered systems
• Many rules and regulations to govern decision making	• Follow agency mission statement and use common sense
• Health and safety is the primary emphasis	• Quality of life in community is the primary emphasis
• Routines are structured for efficiency; activities are done in groups	• Routines are individualized; structured for preferences and new learning
• Specialized treatment services derive from pre-established service categories	• A picture of a better life is created and strategies are designed to make it happen
• Consumer–employee interaction occurs in a congregate setting	• Interaction takes place in the community
• Residents are considered clients or patients needing service	• Residents are considered people who need support to live in the community
• Community 'placement' occurs if the resident demonstrates acceptable skills and behavior	• The person moves to the community and supports and services are built around the person
• The person is seen as a client who needs help and protection	• The person is viewed as a citizen who can make a valuable contribution to society

Table 2. Comparison of clinical problem solving and person-centered planning

Clinical problem solving	Person-centered planning
• Identify deficits, disorders, and problems	• Identify capacities, dreams, and aspirations
• Learn about the person through testing	• Get to know the person informally
• Decision making is hierarchical and professional	• Person, family, and friends decide
• Specialized treatment team meetings	• Group of friends, family, and staff at meetings
• Problems are inside the person	• Problems are in the culture
• Repair the person	• Repair the environment
• The person learns to fit into existing services	• Build supports around the person
• Reduce symptoms	• Enhance quality of life

but this does not mean that it is easier to implement. In addition, Table 2 illustrates the differences of clinical problem solving and person-centered planning.

A COMMENT ABOUT LANGUAGE

Person-centered planners use everyday language. Common language (or plain English) is understood by everyone involved in the planning process. Technical jargon can contribute to the segregation of people with disabilities. For example, *residential program* is replaced with *home, vocational service* with *job,* and *verbal skills* with *talking.* Plain English makes it easier to convey that people with intellectual disabilities have the same basic needs as people without disabilities and enjoy the same basic things in life, including exercising choice, being free of unpleasant conditions, being treated fairly, and having meaningful relationships.

Although person-centered planners try to avoid technical terms in describing the philosophy and practices of person-centered planning, they often use terms that have special meaning and promote social inclusion. For example, words such as *empowerment, citizenship, natural support,* and *building community* have special meaning in the disability field, and they stimulate thinking about how services and supports can be provided toward those ends. We want to make it clear that common language is welcome—even encouraged—so that all people involved in the meeting understand.

Caution: Although person-centered planners use common language, we do not recommend establishing language ground rules in planning meetings. This may stifle discussion and limit the planning process. This caution also holds for agency in-services on person-centered planning. For example, when a speaker who was addressing a group of clinicians insisted that the term *client* was degrading, some audience members contested this premise. After other participants began to defend their own use of the term, the training devolved to an unproductive standoff, which diminished the potential benefit of the training.

COMPARISON OF CLINICAL PROBLEM SOLVING AND PERSON-CENTERED PLANNING

The traditional clinical problem-solving approach entails diagnosing and treating psychopathology. Clinicians typically scan for disorders and impairments and prescribe interventions that prepare the person for the community. Person-centered planning assumes that the person should already be in the community. Here, the problem solving focuses on how to adapt the supports and services to the person in order to maintain quality living in the community. There is overlap between these two approaches. When a person has a medical problem, the clinical method is appropriate (see Pfadt &

Holburn, 1996). As you will see with the PICTURE method, professional services are an inherent part of the process because achieving and maintaining true community inclusion invariably requires professional support.

HOW IS THE PICTURE METHOD DIFFERENT?

Although PICTURE incorporates many aspects of person-centered planning approaches in use today, it attenuates some aspects and adds others. The two main ways in which PICTURE is different are

1. Professionals are welcome. Professional practice is an essential part of the PICTURE method. People with disabilities often have significant physical health and behavioral support needs that require various therapies, interventions, and instructional training that should be provided by people with expert training. However, clinicians, teachers, and other interventionists are encouraged to practice in the community, not in a segregated environment, such as an institution or large group home.

2. Evaluation informs the planners. Throughout the PICTURE process, snapshots of the organization, the individual planning process, and the quality-of-life outcomes are taken periodically in the form of observations, questionnaires, and exercises. Information is fed back to the planning group to guide the planning process and to the management team to maintain organizational support and adaptation. The snapshots are taken in the form of observations, questionnaires, and exercises. These activities reinforce the mission of the organization and the effectiveness of the planning group. Thus, the evaluation tools in PICTURE are more than a measure of effectiveness. They become part of the intervention itself and serve as both process and outcome measures. Members of successful teams that employ the assessments are less inclined to say, "Let's keep doing what we are doing because the evaluation shows it is working" and more apt to say, "Let's keep evaluating because it is getting us where we want to be."

ROLE OF THE PROFESSIONAL IN PICTURE

When I Move into the Community, Who Will Be My Doctor?

Although professional practice is an essential part of the PICTURE process, promoters of person-centered planning are often suspicious of professional services. This caution originates from the history of misapplication of professional treatments in developmental services and the misuse of professional staff in large systems designed to protect and habilitate people with disabilities. However, we believe that such mistreatment is a consequence of poor organizations whose staff have become victims of those systems. Therefore, we believe that professionals, when permitted to practice their trade in the right environment, are not only capable of making a significant contribution to the social inclusion of people with disabilities but are also essential to the process. This is why paid staff are encouraged to participate in PICTURE.

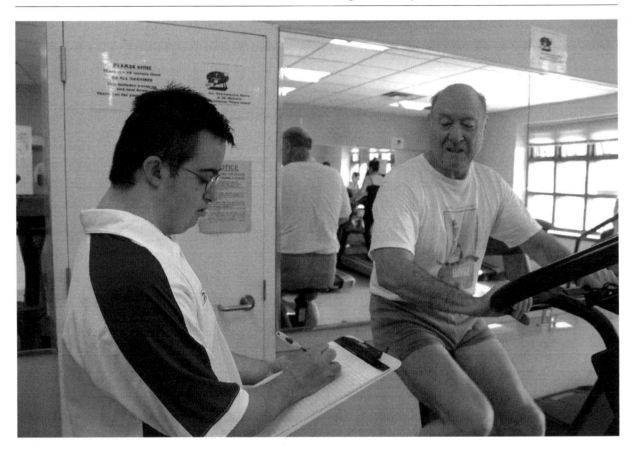

When PICTURE is used, the therapies, teaching, and behavioral interventions take place in the community, not in a segregated environment, such as an institution. Instead of *preparing* individuals to live in the community through various professional practices, the person receives professional treatment in the community. If the person with a disability does not yet live or spend much time in the community, then many services can still be provided in a community neighborhood. Such services include recreation, health care, job development, learning to use public transportation, and behavior support, all of which will bring the professional staff member into the community. Both professionals and individuals with disabilities are participating in the social inclusion process, whereby specialists practice in the community.

An example of the kind of professional practice promoted by PICTURE occurred when changes began to take place at Kessler Avenue Group Home. Twelve individuals live in this home, and they all receive on-site clinical services (i.e., services in the home), including routine medical examinations, as well as speech and physical therapies. The agency management was interested in implementing more person-centered services and began PICTURE meetings with some of the people who live in the Kessler home. One young man, Nolan, who has a variety of medical problems, participated in the PICTURE process. As his planning team was helping him realize his dream to move into an apartment in the community with two friends, Nolan was excited but also apprehensive about the changes that would take place. At one meeting he asked, "When I move into the community, who will be my doctor?" the answer was, "It will be a doctor who practices in the community."

A New Lifestyle Requires New Learning

Teaching is one of the most important activities of the PICTURE approach to person-centered planning. This can include merely the transfer of knowledge or skills to new situations, or it may involve teaching new skills. It is important to teach new skills in the community, rather than teaching them in a segregated setting and hoping that they will generalize to community settings. Team members may be called on to teach these skills or to recruit assistants who will spend time with the person in the community. It is best if agency staff can provide training in the natural environment. For example, if the person with a disability wishes to develop more friends, then he or she may need to learn better ways to talk with people and make friends. Traveling to a new job might require learning how to use public transportation. Living without supervision might mean that the person must learn to cook, clean, and lock the door at night. Many people already have the rudiments of such skills and need relatively little instruction to improve on them and apply them in new circumstances. However, people may initially be reluctant to become more independent and make their own decisions if caregivers have satisfied most of their needs by doing things *for* the person. People with developmental disabilities who have never needed to perform certain tasks will now find themselves needing to learn how to perform them.

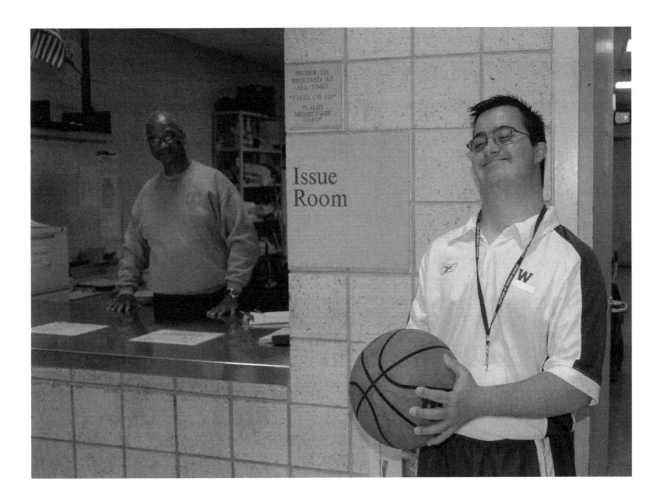

Fostering Friendships

Making friends might be the most important skill for a person who has been excluded from the mainstream of society, but friendship is complex and difficult to define. Nonetheless, a key to inclusion is being able to connect to other people, and people with intellectual disabilities often have difficulty making friends. The disability itself can pose challenges to developing friendships, but people who have lived in segregated settings may have an additional disadvantage because their social development and skills may have been thwarted by lack of opportunity. Some people have opportunities to associate only with staff, family members, or other people with disabilities, but there are many ways to arrange opportunities for friendships to occur.

One way to facilitate friendship is to arrange activities with other people in the community. People who have common interests and talents tend to spend time together talking and sharing ideas. People who work in similar jobs also tend to gravitate toward one another. To the extent that people with disabilities are involved in community life, they are likely to develop friendships with people who live in the community. However, arranging for friendship opportunities is insufficient for many people with disabilities. The development of social skills is needed if the person lacks the repertoire to interact in ways that result in a natural friendship. There is substantial teaching technology in this area, ranging from basic skills such as making eye contact, shaking hands, and reading facial cues, to more complex components comprising appropriate conversation, wearing attractive clothing, and appropriate behavior on a date.

Role of Applied Behavior Analysis and Reinforcement

The most common use of applied behavior analysis is for the reduction of challenging behavior. Interestingly, person-centered planning is often implemented for people with behavior problems, and this is not a coincidence. In fact, the goals and principles of person-centered planning and applied behavior analysis are similar (Holburn, 2001). Person-centered planning can be effective in reducing behavior problems by removing aversive conditions in the person's environment and by providing the person with ready access to reinforcers. The reinforcement in behavior analysis is equivalent to providing access to preferred activities in person-centered planning. Both methods seek to alter what the person does by modifying the environment. Traditional behavior analysis that focuses mainly on eliminating maladaptive behavior does not work in a maladaptive environment. Person-centered planning can be a prerequisite to more successful technical applications of applied behavior analysis by changing the environment so that the person now enjoys where he or she lives or what he or she does.

Sometimes, reinforcers or preferences that are very important to the person are denied by protocol. For example, Brian typically became unmanageable around lunchtime at his day program because he wanted a hot lunch, but the protocol for him and others from his agency was to bring a bag lunch. Consequently, at lunchtime, staff often had to physically contain Brian as they tried to persuade him to enjoy his cold bag lunch, while he observed people from other agencies eating their hot lunches. After considerable red tape, Brian's team arranged for him to have a hot lunch, and his challenging lunchtime behavior disappeared.

Other reinforcers or preferences related to challenging behavior are not so easily obtained. For example, Hal enjoyed visits by his parents so much that the visits were the highlight of his day. However, his mother had stopped visiting him because Hal invariably hit her during the visits. Family visits resumed only after structured behavior analysis sessions with both parents in which Hal was taught to interact more appropriately. This process is described in detail in Holburn and Vietze (2002).

Building on Past Practices and Accomplishments

Person-centered planning should not be promoted as if it were the only way to do things, nor as if everything that preceded it were ineffective. It should not be assumed that a person about to undergo person-centered planning has made no progress. These notions are wrong, and they can repel potential participants. In fact, there is really nothing new about person-centered planning, but its combination of philosophy and practices is unique, and it makes for a powerful method. However, person-centered planning cannot exist in a service vacuum; the planning should be integrated within the organizational culture and process that is currently providing services to the person (Sanderson, 2002). The goals of the person with a disability must be linked to what the person has already accomplished and learned. It is better to build on what is already there than to tear those things down and start over. In this positive approach of PICTURE, we celebrate the skills and achievements already developed and use them as a foundation for further building. This provides continuity and strengthens behaviors that are valued. The solutions that have worked in the past still have value, and they should be acknowledged early on in the planning process.

ASSESSING THE PROCESS AND OUTCOMES

Person-centered planning has the allure of simplicity because the principles are basic and the language is nontechnical, but it is not easy for a planning team to implement the process, nor is it easy for an organization to adjust its structure and procedures in adopting the approach. Thus, another aspect of PICTURE that sets it apart from other methods of person-centered planning is the built-in assessment that guides the process and keeps it on track.

It is not difficult to begin these change processes, but if the team or the larger organization proceeds without evaluating what it set out to do, then it will invariably drift from the new course and end up being pulled back by the processes that governed the team and agency before the person-centered planning was introduced. These influences include regulations, professional practice standards, and the prior conventions of the agency itself, none of which are necessarily counterproductive by themselves. However, in combination, they often produce a rule-governed environment typified by the clinical and bureaucratic processes listed earlier. However, if an agency can keep its eye on the ball of person-centered planning, then the clinical perspective will prevail only with issues of health, and practitioners will apply their skills in ways that advance the person's status as a contributing member of society.

Users of this manual will be able to draw on multiple methods for evaluating each level of implementation: the organization, the planning team, and the person. Each level communicates with the others, and together they function as a unit. The instruments and worksheets on which the evaluation information is based appear in Part IV of this manual. No special training is needed to use the instruments and worksheets, and instructions are provided for their use. It is important to evaluate each level periodically because of the transactional nature of the organizational change process. As change occurs at each level, the changed information is fed back to the planning team and the management team, and that information affects the practices of each team, resulting in new information that is fed back through the cycle. No matter how committed the people are at a single level, their effectiveness hinges on the responsiveness of individuals operating at other levels. Information must be gathered and shared periodically for the components to function as an effective unit. These activities reinforce the mission of the organization and the effectiveness of the planning group. More detailed information about how the PICTURE approach conceptualizes these interlocking functions and how the evaluation and exercises can be used to achieve successful outcomes is provided in Part III.

ELEVEN PRINCIPLES OF PICTURE

1. **People with disabilities should live like people without disabilities.** People with disabilities have the same needs and rights as others in our culture. However, they are often required to live, work, and learn in groups consisting of other people with similar disabilities. If prolonged, this grouping suppresses intellectual and social growth. Furthermore, it can be stigmatizing and degrading, and it usually prevents a person from associating with people without disabilities who live in the community. *PICTURE seeks to remove the stigma and get the person involved with the rest of the main culture, not trapped in a world consisting only of services.*

2. **See the whole person.** Conventional interdisciplinary planning teams consist mostly of professionals and technicians who are responsible for singular aspects of a person's life. For example, the behavior specialist reduces behavior problems, the physical therapist increases range of motion, and the speech-language therapist works on language skills. *PICTURE asks participants not to overfocus on any one aspect of the person. Seeing how one's history, abilities, and aspirations converge to form a picture of a better life requires consideration of many aspects of the person's life, or seeing the person as a whole.*

3. **Individualization.** People with disabilities are often required to undergo daily routines and schedules that do not permit them to pursue their own interests, have choices about what they want to do, or develop their potential. *PICTURE seeks to individualize routines and schedules in ways that promote personal decision making, expand the person's experiences, and develop his or her capacities.*

4. **Natural engagement.** Many people with intellectual disabilities spend much of their time waiting with nothing to do. They are waiting for the bus, the next meal, a therapy session, and so forth. The inactivity results from an unnatural schedule of monotonous activities brought about by the nonindividualized, system-centered way in which many agencies are organized. These extended waiting periods breed boredom and waste

opportunities. *PICTURE seeks to establish a more interesting and productive pattern of activities. The stimulation of preferred opportunities produces a natural engagement in the activities.*

5. **Start where you are; use what you have.** Person-centered planners can be suspicious of service systems and the treatment they provide, but they realize that employees do their best under their given circumstances. Furthermore, the planning cannot take place in a vacuum. To be effective, it needs the input and assistance of professionals who know, serve, and care about the person. *The PICTURE method does not abandon professional services and system components that are consistent with the person-centered approach—it needs them.*

6. **Workers must be helpers.** Employees who assist people with intellectual disabilities begin their careers enthusiastically, excited about helping others. Too often, employees become trapped in bureaucratic roles that remove them from helping roles. *PICTURE seeks to empower the employee to work more constructively and creatively, thus making the relationship more satisfying both to the person with the disability and to the employee.*

7. **Personal commitment.** Person-centered planning is not a mandated or formalized service, and people are rarely hired to do it. Employees are hired to perform certain roles in the organization that hired them. Therefore, the conversion to a person-centered approach means that participants in the planning process will have to do some things outside of their traditional job roles, which requires a personal commitment. *PICTURE's goals are achieved because team members take it on themselves to get the job done.*

8. **Responsive organizations.** Large service systems for people with intellectual disabilities have become industries providing jobs for thousands of employees. Some of these systems have become bureaucracies that are organized in ways that promote the survival of the system over the growth and interests of the people being served. *PICTURE attempts to influence the organization to alter its planning, structure, policies, deployment of staff, allocation of resources, and forms of evaluation to promote person-centered supports and services.*

9. **Bring back the family.** Employees are sometimes uncomfortable when relatives visit the person where he or she lives, works, or goes to school. A father, mother, or other relative might have suggestions and ideas about the care and treatment of their relative, but their ideas might be inconsistent with what the program provides. *PICTURE seeks to give power back to relatives and reunite families who have been disenfranchised and discouraged from maintaining regular contact with their loved one.*

10. **Members of the community must get involved.** Sometimes we are suspicious of the community's interest and ability to provide sufficient health and safety for people with intellectual disabilities. However, many community members are willing and eager to provide help and support, but they rarely even encounter a person with an intellectual disability due to lack of opportunity. *PICTURE facilitates the development of community services and supports for people with disabilities so they can return to their communities. If the person already resides in the community, then the planning team seeks to improve the level of preferred community participation.*

11. **Real friendships are in the community.** People with significant disabilities often have no natural friends with whom they share the same interests. Some people with intellectual disabilities associate only with paid staff and other people with disabilities.

PICTURE recognizes that all people with disabilities have talents and interests that can form the basis of real friendships. *Prerequisite to the development of real friendships, people with disabilities must be exposed to the community, and community members must have contact with people with disabilities.*

PICTURE PRINCIPLES CHECKLIST

The items in this checklist correspond to the PICTURE principles described previously. Think of a person with a disability whom you know or assist, and place a check mark beside the statements that are true. More check marks signify a more person-centered lifestyle. The results can give you an idea of whether he or she would be a good candidate for person-centered planning. They can also be used to identify areas to focus on if the person becomes involved in person-centered planning.

1. _____ The person spends much of his or her time doing things in the community with one or two other people instead of a larger group.

2. _____ The person's planning team discusses ways to make a better life for the person rather than discussing ways to ameliorate deficits and disorders.

3. _____ The person makes choices about important things in life, such as what to do, where to go, and with whom to spend time.

4. _____ The person's activities revolve around his or her interests.

5. _____ The person is receiving services that are helping him or her learn a skill geared toward making a useful contribution to the community.

6. _____ The employees who assist the person are principally engaged in activities that are truly helpful to the person.

7. _____ Employees go outside of their traditional job roles to help the person achieve personal goals.

8. _____ The organization puts the person's needs and interests above the needs of the system.

9. _____ Family members feel welcome to visit the person and are encouraged to give ideas about how things could be better.

10. _____ The person is known in the community and is involved in community activities.

11. _____ The person has friends who live in the community.

PART II

A Step-by-Step Guide

BEFORE YOU BEGIN: KEYS TO SUCCESS

The following factors contribute to the success of the PICTURE process.

Organizational Support

Secure Agency Buy-In

There are many ways to begin person-centered planning in an agency. The process will not be effective if it is imposed from outside on reluctant participants who do not understand it. An appreciation for a more person-centered approach can be gained by staff training, videotapes, circulated written material, and so forth. The agency's state department of mental retardation or developmental disabilities may provide such training materials. An efficient way to learn of resources is through the Internet (see Table 3), although agency executives, managers, direct support staff, clinicians, and other staff should be given an overview of the PICTURE philosophy described in this manual. It is also important for the individuals being served and their family members to feel invested in the process. Initial reactions will range from "We are already doing this" to "We can never do this." We recommend initial training by an outside consultant who is an expert in person-centered planning. Consultants can usually be identified through local informal networks. Table 3 also provides sites that offer training. In any case, understanding new principles and changing the way we do things are never as easy as they seem, but the early attempts to introduce person-centered planning concepts on an agencywide basis will be worth the effort.

Table 3. Internet resources for person-centered planning

Training resource	Internet address
Inclusion Press	www.inclusion.com
Quality Mall	www.qualitymall.org
Community Works	www.communityworks.info
Person Centered Planning Education Site	www.ilr.cornell.edu/ped/tsal/pcp
The Beach Center on Disability	www.beachcenter.org
Capacity Works	www.capacityworks.com
Person-Centered Planning	www.unc.edu/depts/ddti/pages/pcptext.html
Going Far Project	http://www.tash.org/mdnewdirections/index.htm
The Learning Community for Essential Lifestyle Planning	www.elpnet.net

Promote Individualization within the Organizational Culture

In some disabilities agencies, the organizational culture reflects a system approach with very little individualization. This is sometimes called a "cookie cutter" or "one size fits all" approach. Instead of focusing on the person with a disability, the staff, administration, and infrastructure all reflect a culture that is efficient and economical rather than individualized. Even the transportation fleet is a reflection of such a culture, with conspicuous 12- to 15-passenger vans that make moving larger groups of people with disabilities easier. An agency that has such a group culture is not necessarily large, although larger agencies are more likely to provide services in this manner. Person-centered planning, and the PICTURE approach in particular, seeks to modify the organizational culture so that person-centered planning can succeed. Structural and functional changes in the middle and upper levels of the organization are often necessary, requiring direction and support at the highest administrative levels of the organization.

Consider a Community Advisory Board

Because one of the important objectives of person-centered planning is to make connections for people in the community, it is useful for a person-centered agency to have a community advisory board. The purpose of the board is to facilitate community inclusion and to help make things happen for individuals as they become involved in their communities. Board members should be people with influence who are well connected to their own communities and who know about resources that can advance the goals of person-centered planning. Examples of the types of people who might serve on the board are bankers, real estate brokers, recreation leaders, employers, ministers, and business leaders.

These leaders can open doors that strengthen community membership, and they can set examples for others to follow. For example, a manager at a large department store facilitated a job interview for Karen, who has language and writing difficulties and required special assistance to learn the job. Without such support, she would likely not have made it past the application and interview process. A more dramatic example occurred at a community board meeting where a group of neighbors were opposing people with intellectual disabilities living in their neighborhood. Two knowledgeable members of an agency's community advisory board were also in attendance because they anticipated this reaction. They informed the group that property values would not be affected, and gave firsthand accounts of positive attributes of having people with disabilities as neighbors. This testimony was persuasive and effective.

Increase Organizational Capacity to Support Individualized Services

Moving from a *system-oriented* approach to an *individualized* service environment is a commitment the agency must make, even if it has not had the capacity to individualize services in the past. Without this commitment, person-centered planning will flounder. To encourage and support truly individualized services, some agencies must undergo a transformation. The PICTURE method facilitates this process using a reciprocal approach: To support the planning of personalized supports and services, the organization must be informed by the successes and obstacles of the planning groups so as to adjust and maintain organizational support. This manual includes management exercises and instruments to assess the level of person-centeredness in a service agency that can be used as feedback for the organization. More specifically, the PICTURE method provides for a management self-evaluation process in which key members of the management team are able to 1) assess the organizational climate within the agency, 2) evaluate barriers encountered by the person-centered planning teams, and 3) examine their capacity for individualized services against a checklist of organizational indicators that facilitate individualized services (see Part III).

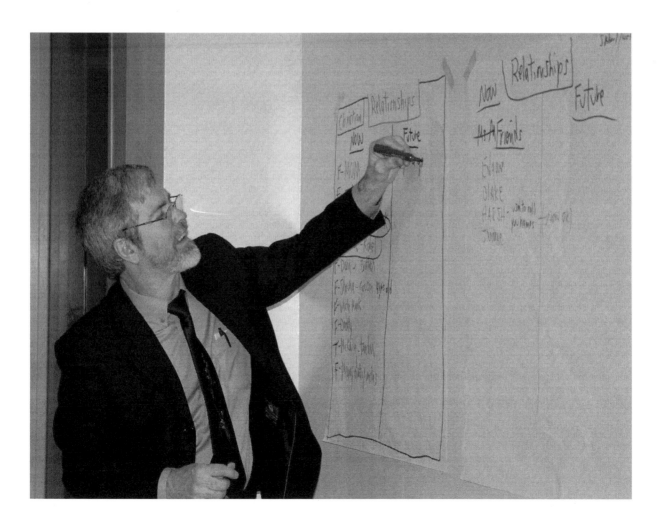

QUALITIES OF A POWERFUL TEAM

An Effective Facilitator

The facilitator is key to the process and in many ways serves as a model for others on the team. He or she organizes and runs meetings and keeps the group focused on core goals and values, such as inclusion, friendships, and personal autonomy. Through consensus, the facilitator helps find ways to accomplish the plan and secures commitments for follow-through. When there are periods of inaction or when the group does not know how to resolve a problem, the facilitator keeps the group together. If the facilitator hangs in there when the going gets tough, then the rest of the team will do the same and group cohesion will be strong. But the facilitator does not do the work alone. With the facilitator modeling optimism and perseverance, other team members will join in the struggle to create a better life for a person. An effective facilitator

- Listens carefully

- Inspires and empowers others

- Promotes collaboration

- Clarifies information

- Stimulates innovation

- Remains flexible

- Stays positive

- Encourages different views

- Reinforces others

We recommend that the facilitator be an agency employee with the requisite skills listed above. Thus, a facilitator could be a social worker, clinician, direct-support worker, or manager. No professional degree or credentials per se are required to facilitate a person-centered planning endeavor.

Using Wall Charts

One of the most important strategies of PICTURE is to chart the plan as it develops. The charts themselves provide a record of the planning process, and they can be used to evaluate progress toward achieving goals for the person with a disability. The charts are important because they make the verbal contributions of the planning team explicit and visible to all team members. When all the charts are hung on the wall, the team can keep in mind the person's interests, the essential elements of the plan, and the steps necessary for achieving the valued outcomes. The charts serve as a kind of group memory. Sometimes patterns emerge from the charts that were not obvious before the charting. As the facilitator systematically constructs a picture of the person's life from the shared information, it is common to hear a team member say, "I never knew that!" The charts can be modified at any time during the process as new information is learned about the person.

Consensus Building

All team members have positive intentions, but they do not always agree. Decisions are reached through discussion and establishment of consensus among team members. Differences might exist, but each member of the group can support the group's collective evaluation, and thus, the decision is generally accepted by members rather than compromised reluctantly. Consensus building is important because the team must work together, and this is the only way the person will be able to achieve his or her goals. As the team struggles to find solutions that permit a high quality of life in the least restrictive setting, issues of risk and safety are ever present and usually require negotiation among team members and with the person with a disability.

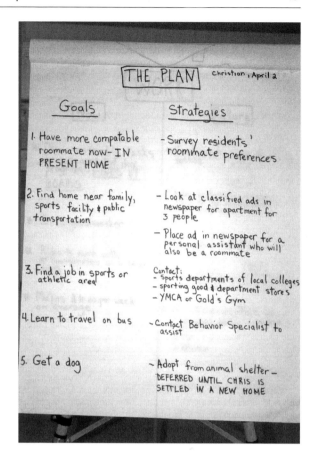

Problem Solving

Person-centered planning is more than getting a group of interested and committed people together and discussing the life and goals of the person. An important ingredient is to be able to solve seemingly unsolvable problems. For example, in our work with Hal, we learned about a major fear felt by his family and the professionals who worked with him. Hal ran fast, and he had a penchant for running across the street without looking for cars. Everyone was afraid that if he went outside, he would run into the street and be injured by a passing car. We discovered that he ran for two reasons: 1) to get to the store across the street and eat candy and 2) because he enjoyed running as an exercise. We reduced the danger by 1) teaching him that if he walked across the street with supervision, he could buy candy at the store; and 2) arranging for him to run regularly at a running track.

Fidelity—Walking the Walk

An essential requirement for any intervention is the degree to which it is implemented according to its specified procedures. Person-centered planning is unique in that it is a complex intervention and it is easy to omit some of the ingredients. When too much of the process is compromised, the person may not realize significant life change. To ensure that the PICTURE process is being implemented appropriately, we have designed two measures to assess the degree to which the planning team and the facilitator are carrying out the process faithfully. These instruments, Assessment of Person-Centered Planning Facilitation and Assessment of Person-Centered Planning Team Integrity, located in Part IV, assess how well the process is being implemented. They can be used to provide feedback to the facilitator and the planning team so that modifications in implementation may be made as the planning proceeds.

SHIFTING CONTROL TO THE PERSON

More Decisions = More Responsibility

Person-centered planning, in which power is transferred from the system to the person with the disability, requires a shift in the thinking of administrators, policy makers, and professionals, who for many years have decided where the person lives, what he or she does, with whom it is done, and at what time. Thus, the first requirement is agency buy-in. An initial step in the planning is acknowledging how much control the employees of the service system have over the life of the person. (The employees of the system are not to blame for this imbalance; it is the way the system is organized, its goals, and the prevailing treatment philosophy that are culpable). However, the shifting of power means that the person will have to take responsibility for his or her decisions. If the person's aspirations threaten his or her health or safety, then negotiation and compromise by team members are in order (see Smull, 1998, and Smull & Lakin, 2002, for a discussion of the competing issues of health and safety, available resources, and what others want for the person).

What Does the Person Really Want?

The first step in promoting decision making by the person with a disability is to encourage the person to give his or her opinion about things. This means that team members must listen to the person when he or she expresses a preference or choice. Consider the idea thoughtfully, rather than dismissing it outright or ignoring it if it sounds unreasonable. If the expressed choice is a clear threat to health or safety, then team members should begin to negotiate alternatives that involve elements of the original idea that are more feasible. Keep the person included in the discussion about alternative ideas, asking him or her for suggestions. If the person is reluctant to participate, then it may be due to his or her inexperience in making decisions, and team members may need to evoke participation slowly and gently. If the person does not understand an issue, then team members should rephrase it in language the person can understand.

Be Respectful

Sometimes we fail to address the person with a disability respectfully. The most basic consideration is that the person should be present during the planning process. During discussion, make eye contact with the person and refrain from talking as if he or she were not present. The person should be addressed as an adult, not as if he or she is a child. It is also important to convey a positive attitude about the person and his or her aspirations. This means that team members believe the person can be successful in his or her pursuits and look ahead toward them, rather than dwelling on how difficult it would be for the person to achieve his or her goals. Obstacles are not ignored; they are acknowledged and addressed in a constructive manner. Another consideration pertains to staying on topic. During difficult problem solving, it is easy to be diverted by tangential comments, so if the conversation begins to drift off topic, the facilitator should guide the conversation back to the person and the purpose of the planning.

Take Periodic Quality Checks

When a team faithfully implements PICTURE, a number of changes tend to occur in the person's life, often at the same time and in different areas. The changes can be fast moving, or they can occur seemingly suddenly after significant planning work. In any case, the progress does not occur in linear fashion. As these changes occur, it is common for successes to create additional challenges that must be overcome. Regular and deliberate assessment of the person's experiences compels team members to take stock of the types and extent of changes that are taking place. The PICTURE method includes measures that permit assessment of the person's quality of life in various life areas, as well as the frequency and types of community activities that the person is experiencing. This information can be used as a guide to evaluate the experiences and address important issues.

CONDUCTING THE MEETINGS: A STEP-BY-STEP GUIDE

Step 1: Get to Know the Person

First Contact

A facilitator who does not yet know the person for whom planning is considered is wise to spend some informal time with the person. These first contacts establish rapport, and they also familiarize the facilitator with the person's life situation. They allow opportunities for people in the life of the person to get to know the facilitator and vice versa.

Conducting the Introductory Meeting

In this meeting, the facilitator describes the PICTURE approach and determines if the person and a few other key players want to participate. A staff person who knows the person well and with whom the person is comfortable should be present. A family member or friend can also be present. In explaining the process, the facilitator describes the purpose of the meetings and the way they are set up, the role of the person, and the benefit that might ensue from the endeavor. After the PICTURE approach is explained, and after the person gives consent to begin the process, the facilitator gleans information for setting up subsequent meetings, such as obtaining background information and identifying who might be interested in being part of the person's planning team. The meeting place atmosphere should be relaxed and without distraction.

1. *Introduce meeting participants.*

2. *Explain the PICTURE approach.* Briefly describe the philosophy and approach of person-centered planning, and discuss the differences between person-centered planning and conventional planning, highlighting key points such as individualized services, decision making, and community membership. Describe what happens at person-centered planning meetings versus conventional meetings, contrasting the different qualities of each.

3. *Gather preliminary information.* Discuss the person's routines and activities and encourage him or her to share one or two wishes or dreams for the future. This discussion will help the person understand the purpose of the planning meetings, and it will help the facilitator plan the sequence of charts to use at the first planning meeting.

4. *Identify team members.* Generally, a team that is composed of a diverse group of people who are interested in making a difference in the life of the person can produce significant consequences. Ideally, the team should consist of the facilitator, the person with a disability, family members, friends (e.g., peers, neighbors, other individuals in the community), interested clinicians, and other preferred agency employees such as support staff. When considering whom to invite, keep in mind that creative thinking, knowledge of community resources, and knowledge of family resources are valuable qualities. Get names, contact information, and other details that might be helpful.

5. *Consider cofacilitation.* It may be useful to have a cofacilitator who is a member of the person-centered team and an employee of the agency. This can be planned ahead of time so that the facilitator mentors the cofacilitator throughout the process. In this way, the cofacilitator can assume the full facilitator role without interrupting the process.

6. *Plan the next meeting.* Determine the time and place for the meeting or identify tentative times and places to be confirmed later. The meeting can be held almost anywhere, including a location at the agency assisting the person. A location in the community sends a strong inclusion message. As the planning proceeds, meeting venues can change. For example, with Hal, initial meetings were held at his parents' home, and subsequent meetings occurred at his primary agency, as well as prospective agency day programs and community residences.

7. *Planning after the meeting.* When inviting potential team members to participate, be sure to articulate the general approach, goals, and processes of person-centered planning. If possible, the person can write out and send invitations, by regular mail or email, including the time and location of the meeting. Consider an RSVP. It is also a good idea to send prospective team members information about the PICTURE method.

Facilitator Tips: Arranging the Life Picture Meeting

A good deal of up-front work is required in setting the stage for a productive person-centered planning meeting. The following will make for a strong beginning:

- *The person.* The person should attend. Make sure the date and time are arranged for convenience of the person.

- *Location.* Hold the meeting in a location with enough space and room for wall charts. It should be private enough for the person and team members to feel comfortable in speaking freely about personal issues. Meetings that are held away from the agency minimize disruptions and may facilitate new ideas.

- *Seating.* Encourage participation of the person, family members, and other nonagency attendees by having them sit up front. Wall charts should be visible.

- *Refreshments.* This might not sound like an essential ingredient for planning lifestyle changes, but having food and drink available sends a message to participants. It contributes to a relaxed atmosphere and enhances the social process.

- *Charting materials.* Charting is inherent to PICTURE and especially important in the early planning stages. Recording important points with markers on flip-chart paper improves communication and problem solving. The charts can be displayed at later meetings for continuity, clarification, and reflection on the planning process and outcomes.

- *Assemble a powerful team.* Try to stack the deck with people who are willing to work toward a significant change for the person, including the person, family members, friends, pertinent staff members, and others who could add to the planning or implementation. If all attendees are agency employees, then the process may resemble an interdisciplinary team meeting.

Step 2: Develop Pictures of the Present and Future

A Whole View of the Person

The PICTURE method of person-centered planning focuses on improving the life of a person with a developmental disability by first developing pictures of eight quality-of-life aspects of his or her life.

1. Relationships

2. Home life

3. Work, school, or day activity

4. Community places

5. Community competence

6. Respect

7. Physical and behavioral health

8. Preferences and choices

The pictures appear as wall charts created from information provided by the group during meetings that are led by a facilitator. Each of the eight charts is divided in two. One side reflects the person's life as it is now; the other side reflects the dreams and hopes of how life might look in the future. It is likely that life changes will not be desired for each of the eight quality-of-life areas, but we recommend reviewing each area to get a whole view of the person.

Developing the present and future life pictures might take more than one meeting, and some pictures will receive more emphasis than others (see Figure 1). As information is added, a view of the person's life unfolds in a way that has not been synthesized and displayed before. It becomes clear to everyone involved how the person's life could be made better, and it is at this point in the planning that the group begins to develop a common purpose and the motivation to work together.

Information is recorded on large pieces of paper that everybody can see to facilitate group cohesion and enhance the planning in general. Common flip-chart paper or other paper that can be taped to a wall is sufficient. Large, multicolored markers are used to designate themes or contrasts that can be helpful to the person and the rest of the team. For example, it can be revealing to record undesirable aspects in red, desirable aspects in green, and neutral content in blue or black. The facilitator has a complex task of asking questions, listening, encouraging participation, and recording responses on the chart paper.

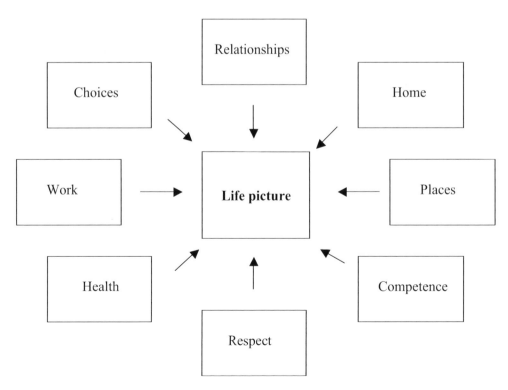

Figure 1.   Life picture.

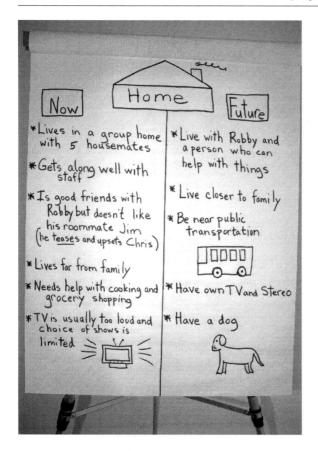

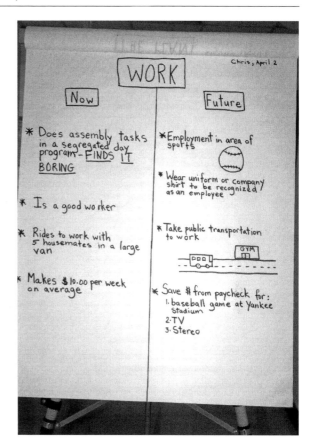

Conducting the Life Picture Meeting

1. *Introduce team members.* It's important for team members to be comfortable with one another. They will be meeting in the future to clarify the person's aspirations and will work together to make those aspirations become a reality through consensus, group problem solving, and follow-through responsibilities.

2. *Explain the purpose of the meeting.* As was done in the first meeting, briefly describe the philosophy and approach of person-centered planning, and discuss key differences between person-centered planning and conventional planning.

3. *Compose ground rules.* This is an important step, and it is not difficult. Engage the group in suggesting rules that will enhance discussion and problem solving, and write them on a wall chart. (The rules may remain visible at initial meetings and might need to be reviewed and displayed at selected follow-up meetings.) The facilitator can begin the exercise by offering the first rules, or the team may generate all or some of them. Because consensus is required, this is the first time members will interact as a group. Suggested ground rules are as follows.

   - Keep the person's interests and wishes at the center of the discussion.

   - Listen to others' perspectives.

   - Think and speak positively.

   - Allow only one person at a time to speak; limit side conversations.

   - Be sensitive to others' feelings when offering information.

- Be patient and respectful of everyone's words and ideas, especially those of the person.

4. Develop the *present* life picture of the first quality-of-life aspect (see Figure 2). The facilitator gathers information from the person and other team members that describes the person's life as it is now. The present life situation becomes a reference, or starting point, for the team to envision a better quality of life for the person.

Start with the relationships picture. Write *Relationships* at the top of the page and separate the page in half by making a vertical line down the center. Label the column on the left *Life as It Is Now* (or similar title). Record each person's name and their role in the life of the person. The amount of detail depends on how many people are involved in the life of the person. (Be sure to include meeting participants, even if they are not significant to the person at present.)

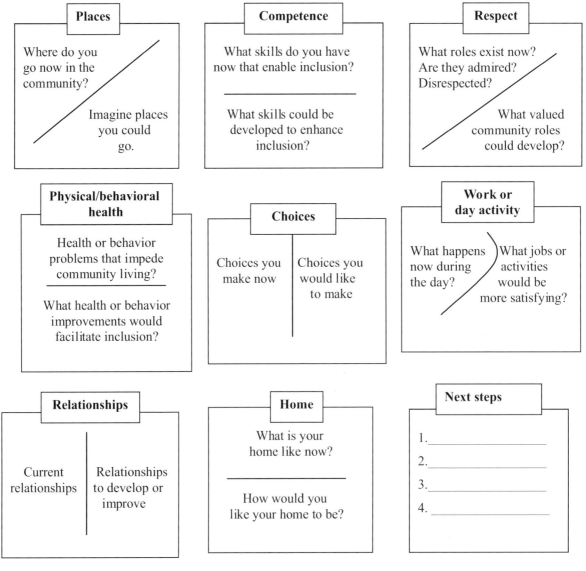

Figure 2. Present and future PICTURES.

A note about the *Choices* chart: The *Choices* chart is the most versatile chart in PICTURE. It can be used early in the process to illuminate what the person enjoys most in life, and what he or she can do well. It also can be introduced last as a means of identifying other interests that might have been missed in the process. Thus, depending on a person's situation and the course of the charting process, *Choices* allows the facilitator to chart contrasts such as (a) *Things I Like to Do* versus *Things I Want to Do More of,* (b) *Things I Like* versus *Things I Dislike,* and (c) *Choices I Have Now* versus *Choices I Would Like to Make.* Much of the content in the *Choices* chart will overlap with content from the other charts, and this redundancy will tend to highlight the most important features of the future PICTURE for the person.

5. Next, develop the *future* life picture of the first quality-of-life aspect. In this step, the facilitator encourages the team to be mindful of the dreams and aspirations of the person and to be innovative in imagining a future life. It is not necessary at this point to get a complete picture of how life could be better in each of the eight aspects; this information can be filled in as the planning proceeds.

   After recording the person's current relationships, develop a picture of what future relationships might be like. For example, for future relationships, the person may wish to have a different roommate, find a girlfriend, reestablish a relationship with a long-lost relative, or spend more time with an existing friend. Record the future picture on the other side of the chart under a heading such as *Life as It Could Be* (or similar title).

6. Repeat steps 4 and 5 for the remainder of the quality-of-life aspects. For guidance in charting each of the eight quality-of-life aspects, see the section titled Suggested Questions for Developing Life Pictures. More than one meeting might be needed to complete this step.

7. Summarize the present and future pictures. Before concluding the meeting, review each picture. During this summary, clarify cloudy or ill-defined issues, and encourage members to offer additional information for the charts. Remind the group that more information can be added later.

8. Introduce the evaluation component. Briefly review the rationale and process of evaluating

Who	What	When
Rosalee (house manager)	Talk to residents to find out their roommate preferences and make room changes if possible	starting tomorrow
Chris & Melvin (favorite worker)	Buy Sunday newspaper and circle possible apartments	Next Sunday
Melvin	Make appointments for Chris and him to visit apartments	End of next week
Chris & Daniel (brother)	Visit Wagner College Sports Dept. about job or volunteer possibilities	by April 17th
Chris & Melvin	Ask managers of Modell's, Sears, the YMCA, and Gold's gym about employment or volunteering	by End of Month
Tina (behavior specialist)	Take Chris on a bus to determine learning needs	by April 30th

the organization, planning team, and the personal outcomes, as delineated in Part IV of the manual. At this point, a few assessments can be described, but this is not the time to describe or plan the administration of the instruments.

9. Determine actions that need to be taken for the next meeting. It might be wise to invite new members to become part of the team at this point, but in general, there should not be much follow-up needed for developing the life picture. However, immediate needs for follow-through might become apparent during discussion, and now is the time to clarify action needed, who is responsible, and when it is expected to be completed. This information should be recorded on a chart titled *Next Steps* (see Figure 2).

10. Set the date, time, and location of the next meeting with the team. The next meeting might be a continuation of developing the life picture.

The following questions are designed to stimulate thinking and discussion about life as it is now and how it could be better. Some questions pertain to more than one quality-of-life aspect.

Suggested Questions for Developing Life Pictures

Relationships

- With whom does the person live?

- With whom does he or she work, participate in day activities, or go to school?

- Who is in the family? Which family members are involved in the person's life?

- Who in the community does he or she have contact with? Who are his or her friends?

- Who are the staff people with whom he or she has the most contact?

- Whom does he or she get along with? Whom does he or she dislike?

- Who helps her or him? Whom does he or she help?

- Are there relationships that should be strengthened or discontinued?

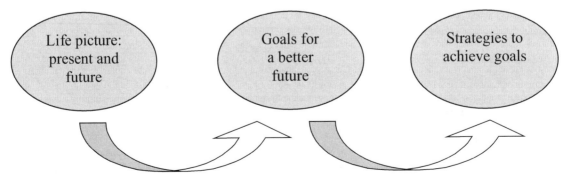

Figure 3.   Life pictures/goals/strategies.

Home

- If the person lives in an agency residence, does he or she get along with house-mates and residential staff members?

- If the person lives at home with the family, what is the quality of the family relationships?

- Is the home well maintained? Is the neighborhood safe?

- Is there enough space for privacy?

- Does he or she like the home?

- Is it convenient for shopping, restaurants, houses of worship, and so forth?

- Does he or she participate in the upkeep of the home in some way?

- Does the person choose which chores to do or when to do them?

Work, School, or Day Activity

- Is the physical environment clean and well maintained?

- Does the outside of the building call negative attention to itself for any reason?

- Are peers, co-workers, and staff friendly and supportive?

- Is there interaction with people without disabilities?

- Is the workplace, school, or day program segregated from the community?

- If the person does not have a job, then can the person volunteer?

- Are there educational or training opportunities that promote growth and advancement?

- Does the job, school, or day activity create a sense of worth and pride in the person?

Community Places

- Where and how often does the person go to church, a ball game, bowling, swimming, the movies, the park, a museum, a picnic, or a play in the community?

- Where does he or she like to go? Dislike to go?

- How often does the person visit a grocery store, shopping mall, hairdresser, bank, or restaurant?

- What is the mode of transportation? Does anyone accompany the person?

- Does he or she have money to spend?

- Does he or she visit friends or family members in the community?

- How can he or she have greater opportunity to experience new places and visit more places that are preferred?

Community Competence

- Is the person learning skills that will lead to a meaningful job or social role? Will these skills facilitate becoming a productive member of the community?

- What kind of interaction occurs with people at the store, movies, concerts, museums, health club, library, and so forth?

- Does he or she receive training to improve personal care, communication, or social interaction?

- Is the person learning skills that enhance his or her chances of moving to or remaining in the community?

- Are opportunities provided to practice skills?

- Are there opportunities to make wants and needs known?

- Does the person need formal job development training?

Respect

- Do the person's environment and activities promote dignity and respect, or are these factors stigmatizing?

- Does he or she travel in a large group in which most of the members have disabilities?

- Does the person ride to work, school, or other activities in a van with the agency name conspicuously displayed on it?

- Are clean, fashionable clothes worn?

- Does the person's behavior set him or her apart from others?

- Does the person's job make a contribution to society?

- Is he or she enrolled in a school or training program leading toward that goal?

Physical and Behavioral Health

- Can he or she choose a doctor? Does he or she have a good relationship with the doctor?

- Is medication taken independently or with assistance? Is there a problem with the medication?

- Does he or she exercise and eat healthfully?

- How often does the person participate in preferred activities that promote health and well-being?

- Does he or she have adequate access to health care and behavioral support?

- If the person has challenging behavior, is applied behavior analysis or behavior therapy used to address the behavior?

Preferences and Choices

- If employed, does the person enjoy the job? How was this occupation chosen?

- Is the person satisfied with his or her living arrangements? If not, does he or she have the power to change them?

- What are the person's favorite things to do?

- What hobbies, talents, and interests would the person like to pursue or do more of?

- Who shops for groceries? Does the person get to eat meals that he or she likes?

Facilitator Tips: Facilitating the Life Picture Meeting

Much of the strength and cohesion of the person-centered team depends on the facilitator. More than any other team member, the facilitator organizes the planning process, keeps the team together, and reinforces team member efforts and accomplishments.

- *Why are we here?* At the very beginning of the meeting, briefly state the purpose of the gathering and what the group will be doing. Because the process evolves, it is important to summarize the purpose of each meeting to orient participants.

- *Review prior commitments.* Early in the meeting, review pending strategies and action steps, and ask participants to report on what they said they would do.

- *Uncover the details.* Bring out important and often overlooked information about the life of the person. Ask probing questions beginning with "what," "why," "where," and "when." For example, instead of asking, "Does she like to watch movies?" ask, "What does she like to do?"

- *Keep the person in focus.* When discussion drifts, redirect it toward the interests and desires of the person. If there is disagreement about what the group should be working toward, then refocus on what the *person* wants. Negotiation might be necessary to balance aspirations with health and safety.

- *Build instead of repair.* To enhance quality of life in the community, solicit information about the person's strengths, abilities, and interests related to community living, rather than identifying deficits to be ameliorated. Bring professional skills to bear on obstacles such as taking the bus, making friends, getting a job, and other ways to enhance community inclusion.

- *Use wall charts.* Record team member contributions on charts that everyone can see, and summarize them occasionally during the meeting. This information increases understanding and helps maintain focus during the meeting.

- *Clarify responsibilities.* When a team member makes a commitment to take action, restate or clarify the strategy, document the action to be taken, and identify the time frame for achievement of the action.

- *Summarize the action plan.* As the meeting concludes, remind team members of their commitments, preferably using the charts as a reference. Review the action steps by restating each strategy, the person responsible for carrying it out, and the time frame.

- *Keep a record.* Written documentation, such as wall charts or notes, should occur as the meeting proceeds. The record preserves the history of the group, and it can be forwarded to team members for follow-up.

- Who decides on clothing? Who shops for clothing?

- Who decides on a bedtime? When to eat?

- Can the person decide who to spend his or her time with?

- Are the person's desires, preferences, and interests taken into account in decisions that others make for him or her?

Step 3: Plan a Better Future

In this step, the team 1) reviews the future life pictures, 2) determines what parts of the future life pictures should become goals to work toward, and 3) develops strategies to accomplish the goals (See Figure 4).

Developing the Plan for a Better Future

1. Redisplay and review the completed life picture (eight life areas; present and future).

2. Determine which future images or ideas from the life picture should become goals. Here, the facilitator helps the team decide which aspirations to work toward and converts those images into goals. Images to be developed into goals can be starred or underlined by the facilitator. Record the goals on the *Plan for a Better Future* chart located below. Remember, planning is a continuous process; decisions made during the meeting are not permanent. Ideas that are not included now can be reconsidered at a later time.

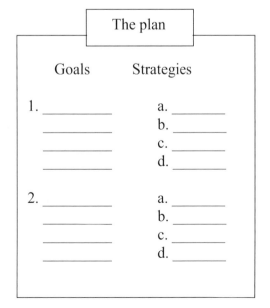

Figure 4.   Plan for a better future and next steps chart.

3. Prioritize the goals. Prioritize goals on the basis of the person's needs, capabilities, interests, desires, and complexity of the goal. Some goals may emerge as needing attention as soon as possible. Some goals will be easy to accomplish, such as purchasing an alarm clock to get to work on time. Still others will require sustained effort, with multiple steps and strategies. Achieving goals, no matter how small, has a cumulative effect on group cohesion. Seeing the person experience positive changes during the process motivates team members to continue to work together to accomplish more parts of the unfinished future life picture.

4. Brainstorm strategies to achieve the goals. Here, team members discuss ways to accomplish the goals. Record these strategies on the *Plan for a Better Future* chart (see Figure 4) located in this section. These charts may get a bit messy because they are a work in progress. Some ideas for strategies may be added or deleted after discussion.

5. Develop next steps. Identify volunteers to carry out strategies and tasks. On the *Next Steps* chart (See Figure 4), record 1) *who* will be responsible for the task, 2) *what* the person will do, and 3) *when* the task will be completed. The *Next Steps* chart will be completed over the course of the meeting as suggestions emerge for actions to be taken. If additional people are needed to help implement the plan, such as experts in a certain area, then they can be invited to the next meeting.

6. Summarize the goals, strategies, and next steps. The facilitator reviews what the team has agreed to as the plan for a better future, which consists of the goals, strategies, and responsibilities of team members. Make sure everyone understands and agrees to their commitments. This step tends to confirm consensus. At this point, vague issues come to the forefront that require clarification and possible strategy modification.

7. Establish a date, time, and place for the next meeting. Be sure that the date for the next meeting corresponds to the time frames listed on the *Next Steps* chart.

Step 4: Implement the Plan

So far, this manual has described the philosophy of the PICTURE method and the development of a person's plan for a better future. Step 4 of the process entails follow-through activities that occur *between* meetings. This is where the real work of person-centered planning takes place, including teaching new skills and employing the evaluation components of PICTURE. The follow-through activities determine whether the team will be successful in achieving the goals. Team members must follow through with their responsibilities outlined in the *Next Steps* chart. At follow-through meetings, team members report their activities and progress, and strategies are altered as necessary. New goals often develop as a consequence of discussion at follow-through meetings.

Facilitator Tips: Problem Solving During PICTURE Meetings

Significant change does not occur without problem solving, which begins when the team has a clear picture of the future. The degree of problem solving required is proportional to the difference between the person's present situation and the person's idea of a better future. In other words, bigger changes call for more problem solving. Figuring out how to overcome obstacles is the heart of the PICTURE process. The suggestions that follow will increase the chances of discovering effective solutions.

- *Stay positive!* The facilitator's confidence can be contagious and uplifting, especially when challenges appear insurmountable or when there are droughts of inaction in implementation. At such times, remind members of their accomplishments and the significance of their mission. Making the future picture become a reality entails occasional disappointments, which are buffered with a positive attitude.

- *Get everyone's input.* People will be invested in the change process if they are involved in the discussion. To assure participation, ask each team member to give their opinion on a particular issue or give their impression of the meeting before it concludes. If the person with a disability cannot communicate clearly, then others who are knowledgeable about the person should present his or her preferences.

- *Clarify vague information.* Team members will need clarification when terms or acronyms are unclear. Restate these in plain English. Complex issues are made clearer by charting key points on wall charts, which contributes to problem solving.

- *Obtain consensus.* Solutions should reflect members' shared ideas, including those of the person. When the team confronts a difficult issue, be sure the problem is clear to the group and clarify different perspectives on how to resolve it. Wall charts can illustrate pros and cons. Select the strategy that is acceptable to most team members.

- *Don't get bogged down with system obstacles.* Address system constraints when policies, structure, or lack of resources appears to prevent moving forward, but avoid prolonged discussion of impediments to achievement. Redirect such discussion to alternative approaches that might accommodate the goals.

- *Reinforce participation.* Give positive feedback when team members share information and ideas that contribute to the process of creating a better life for the person.

- *Encourage innovation.* A can-do attitude supplemented with creative thinking helps overcome obstacles and facilitates implementation of the plan. Encourage team members to think "outside the box" and brainstorm possible solutions without criticism.

Conducting Follow-Through Meetings

Follow-through meetings begin after the plan for a better future has been developed. The follow-through meetings consist mostly of problem-solving discussions about the plan's implementation.

1. *Review strategies and commitments.* The facilitator displays and reviews with the team the charts that list goals, strategies, and next steps.

2. *Report on progress and obstacles to the goals.* Team members discuss progress made and barriers encountered while carrying out the plan strategies. The facilitator can record this information using the format (or similar one) shown on the *Problem Solving* chart shown in this section. Displaying the strategies that are working well

and the problems that are encountered will help the team form a clearer picture of how to proceed. This information can also be used as a record of meeting proceedings.

3. *Evaluate process and outcomes.* Follow-through meetings are the context for periodic reporting of the evaluation results. Exercises for the planning team, described in the next section, can constitute significant portions of follow-through meetings in providing feedback to the team on 1) how faithfully it is adhering to the PICTURE process and 2) what the person has been experiencing since it began.

4. *Alter goals and strategies as needed.* Goals are altered or added and strategies are adjusted to accommodate new information or changing circumstances. New information is added to the life picture as it emerges. New goals and strategies can be recorded on the original charts or on a new chart using the format (or similar one) shown on the *Revising the Plan* chart (see Figure 5).

5. *Determine next steps on the basis of progress that has been made, and record them on the original* Next Steps *charts as a continuation of prior steps or on a new* Next Steps *chart.*

Promoting Follow-Through

The following suggestions will help maintain planning momentum between meetings and increase the likelihood of accomplishing the goals.

1. *Photograph and distribute charts.* Charts showing goals, strategies, and next steps can be easily duplicated with a digital camera and computer equipment and distributed as reminders to team members.

2. *Make telephone calls to people who have volunteered to take action.* Calls can be made by the facilitator or a volunteer from the team to members to see how things are going. Problem solving may be needed during telephone calls if tasks cannot be completed as originally planned or if unexpected issues arise.

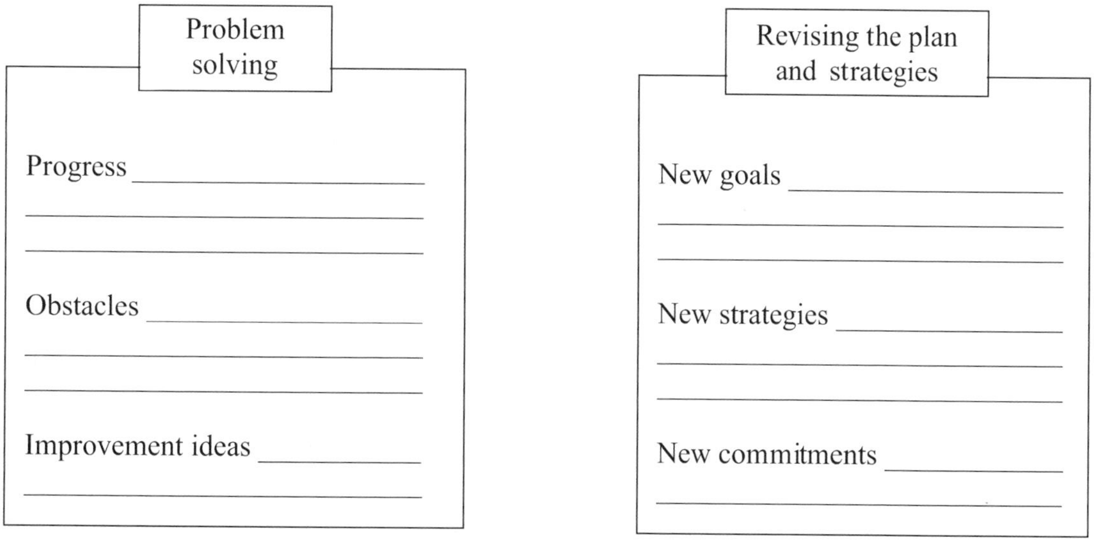

Problem solving	Revising the plan and strategies
Progress _____ _____ _____	New goals _____ _____ _____
Obstacles _____ _____ _____	New strategies _____ _____ _____
Improvement ideas _____ _____	New commitments _____ _____

Figure 5.   Problem solving and revising the plan charts.

3. *Remind team members of the next meeting.* Any form of notice will do, including telephone calls, letters, or e-mail. A simple reminder sent a few days before the meeting can increase attendance.

4. *Hold regular meetings.* Some facilitators maintain group cohesion and momentum by holding meetings on a regular basis (e.g., one per month). If too much time elapses between meetings, then the team will have a lot of catching up to do.

5. *Maintain team identity.* Distinguish PICTURE meetings from the conventional interdisciplinary team meetings in which deficit-oriented program plans are reviewed. Because of the different format, goals, and purposes of the two types of processes, attempts to combine the two meetings are likely to result in diluting rather than strengthening the PICTURE process.

6. *Establish subcommittees.* Sometimes a complex issue is best dealt with by forming small ad hoc groups that meet between follow-through meetings to resolve a problem or learn more about the issue. Subcommittees can also serve to plan and organize components of the evaluation that the team will use for feedback.

PART III

Using Evaluation to Improve the PICTURE

EVALUATING THE PERSON, TEAM, AND ORGANIZATION

Person-centered planning will be successful if the organization, team, and the individual are communicating and operating as a unit. These three components are displayed below as a general framework for conceptualizing the PICTURE process. As Figure 6 suggests, the process is transactional in that each component is influenced by the other two.

In this model of person-centered planning within an agency, the organization generates a person-centered process for an individual whose experiences influence the individual planning process, both of which are fed back to the organization, which must adjust its practices to further accommodate the person-centered process for that individual. It is recognized that the first two components are not mutually exclusive because there occasionally is some overlap in 1) membership of organizational team and 2) their functions in planning for and assisting the person. Similarly, the sequences of influence may not be as clear as they are depicted in the figure. For example, the organizational support may directly influence the person and vice versa.

Person-centered planning cannot thrive in an agency that does not continually adapt to the individual. The organization and the larger system of which it is a part must promote the person-centered philosophy and support its practices, yet the organization must be guided by the very process it advocates. Therefore, the practices of the organization must change to sustain true individualization. These changes might entail alter-

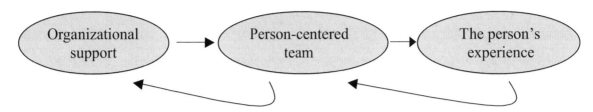

Figure 6. Organizational support, person-centered team, the person's experiences.

ations of funding sources, staff deployment, training, methods of transportation, hiring practices, job descriptions, and so forth.

In the PICTURE method, these three areas of interlocking function are assessed using the instruments and worksheets presented in Part IV of the manual. They render information that is fed back to members of the person-centered planning team, as well as to individuals providing organizational support. The different ways in which the information is applied are described in the following exercises. It is not necessary to use all of the instruments and worksheets, but it is recommended to address each of the three components so that the organization, team, and individual operate together as an effective unit.

The Person's Experiences

1. An assessment of the person's quality of life is measured by the Person-Centered Planning Quality-of-Life Indicators (Holburn, Pfadt, Vietze, Schwartz, & Jacobson, 1996), which assess eight areas of outcome associated with the PICTURE planning process. These assessed areas correspond to the eight areas constituting the life picture.

2. A snapshot of the person's community involvement during a 14-day period is taken with the Community Activities Checklist (adapted from Kennedy et al., 1990), which indicates for each activity 1) its type, 2) the degree of support needed, and 3) whether the experience was enjoyable.

3. An evaluation of how satisfied the person is with his or her degree of input into the PICTURE planning process, and with his or her life in general, is determined from the Decision Making and Satisfaction Interview (Holburn, Gordon, & Vietze, 2006).

Person-Centered Planning Team Process

1. An evaluation of how faithfully the facilitator conducts the planning process is made by an independent observer who attends meetings and completes the Assessment of Person-Centered Planning Facilitation Integrity form (Holburn, Gordon, & Vietze, 2001, see Part IV for form).

2. The degree of group cohesion and person-centeredness among team members is evaluated with the Assessment of Person-Centered Planning Team Integrity form (Holburn, Vietze, Jacobson, & Gordon, 2003a, see Part IV). This observational measure reflects team interaction during person-centered planning meetings.

3. An assessment of how consistently the team is adhering to the principles of PICTURE described earlier is conducted using the Eleven Principles of PICTURE: What is Our Team Working Toward? worksheet. This measure can be especially useful for problem solving when the team has hit a roadblock or for clarifying and renewing its mission if the team has drifted off track in its planning process.

Organizational Support

1. The degree to which staff members feel that a person-centered atmosphere prevails in an agency is measured with the Person-Centered Organizational Climate Survey (Holburn, Vietze, Jacobson, & Gordon, 2003b). This is an anonymous survey that permits the management team to evaluate overall agency climate and possible differences between organizational divisions and between disciplines.

2. The management team can efficiently identify obstacles to the person-centered planning teams by reviewing the Barriers to Plan Implementation Form (Holburn & Gordon, 2003), which lists organizational impediments (e.g., policy, training, resources, staffing) to the goals established by the teams. Barriers are listed in categories that correspond to the eight areas constituting the life picture.

3. A global perspective on the fit between what the agency offers to people with disabilities and what the agency provides to foster quality of life outcomes can be ascertained using the Relationship Between the Organization and Quality-of-Life Outcomes worksheet as a discussion guide.

4. Person-Centered Organizational Capacity Indicators is a checklist of factors that increase the organization's capacity for individualized services that yield person-centered outcomes. This checklist suggests 19 ways in which the organization can yield these outcomes.

EXERCISES FOR THE PLANNING TEAM

The team process is an intervention that attempts to make significant improvements in the life of the person with a disability (see Figure 7 for an illustration of this process). It is especially important to evaluate what the team actually does in carrying out person-centered planning because of the multiple components involved. This process is evaluated by examining the performance of the facilitator, the interaction of the team, and adherence to the principles of the PICTURE method. The person's experiences (i.e., personal outcomes) are assessed by evaluating his or her quality of life, community

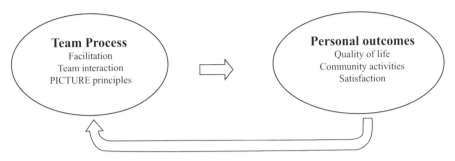

Figure 7.   Team process and personal outcomes chart.

participation, and level of decision making and satisfaction. All of this information can be fed back to the team for analysis and modification of the process so that it truly facilitates a better life for the person.

The following exercises describe ways to increase the strength of the planning team in creating a better lifestyle for the person. When the person is incorporated into the team process, he or she becomes an aspect of the intervention itself. In addition, the person also evaluates the effectiveness of the intervention—this is what we mean when we say the evaluation serves both the process and the outcome of PICTURE. Thus, the exercises usually occur as part of the person-centered planning meetings.

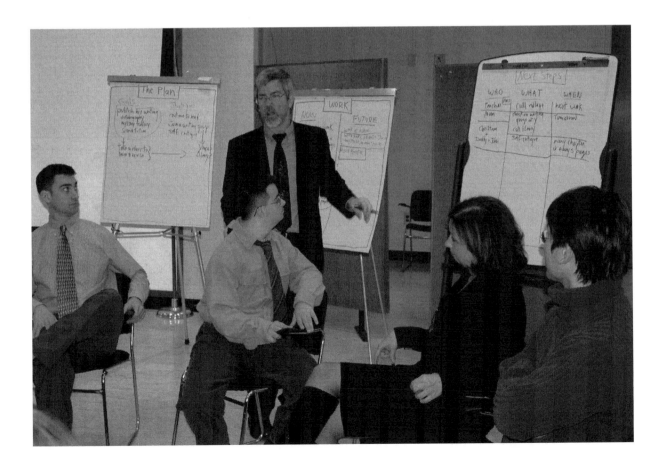

Planning Team Exercise 1:
Taking a Look at Overall Quality of Life

> **Purpose:** This exercise is intended to inform team members about various aspects of life the person is experiencing and to suggest areas for improvement.

Information source: Person-Centered Planning Quality-of-Life Indicators

How to obtain the information: The survey can be completed by an independent evaluator, team members, or one team member designee. The person with a disability should give input if possible.

How to evaluate and use the feedback: Results for the eight quality of life areas are reviewed and discussed with all team members, including the person. Selected areas can be evaluated item by item. The results can be used to establish new goals, to augment existing goals and strategies, and to evaluate team progress.

Planning Team Exercise 2:
Increasing Community Participation

> **Purpose:** To identify the types and frequencies of community activities the person experiences, including the level of support needed. This exercise can be used to develop a richer schedule of preferred community activities.

Information source: Community Activities Checklist

How to obtain the information: The checklist is completed outside of the planning meeting by someone who knows about the person's daily activities. This survey can be completed by an independent evaluator, team members, or one team member designee. The person with a disability should give input if possible. Additional activities can be added to the form.

How to evaluate and use the feedback: The results are shared with the team during a planning meeting. They can be used to strengthen community participation by highlighting additional activities to schedule and by evaluating the degree of support needed and the preference level for the different activities. Team members may wish to use the checklist as a basis for developing a list of available local community activities. The person or designee should be at the meeting to give input about preferences and to report new or recent community activities experienced.

Planning Team Exercise 3:
Keeping the Focus on the Person

> **Purpose:** To find out how the person feels about his or her involvement in the PICTURE planning process and the extent to which the team is working toward life goals most important to the person.

Information source: Decision Making and Satisfaction Interview

How to obtain the information: Information is derived through an interview conducted with the person with a disability, including his or her parents or advocate, as appropriate.

How to evaluate and use the feedback: With permission, the interviewer shares the information with planning team members. Accordingly, the facilitator and team may need to adjust their strategy to correspond with the person's level of decision making and life areas in which he or she deems most important.

Planning Team Exercise 4:
Conducting a Person-Centered Planning Meeting

> **Purpose:** To maintain facilitation integrity (proper implementation) of person-centered planning meetings according to the PICTURE facilitator guidelines.

Information source: Assessment of Person-Centered Planning Facilitation Integrity

How to obtain the information: This checklist is completed after the meeting by an independent observer, who must pay careful attention to the definitions and criteria for items (see instructions located in Part IV). This checklist should also be used as part of the facilitator's training, so the facilitator should be aware of the criteria for satisfying each item.

How to evaluate and use the feedback: The results are shared with the facilitator in a private meeting. This feedback can help guide the facilitator in maintaining fidelity of the facilitation.

Planning Team Exercise 5:
How Person-Centered Is Our Planning Team?

> **Purpose:** To determine the degree of person-centered interaction during planning meetings and raise consciousness among members.

Information source: Assessment of Person-Centered Planning Team Integrity

How to obtain the information: This rating scale is completed by an independent observer who completes the rating scale after the meeting (see instructions located in

Part IV). Prior to this team assessment, team members should have received fundamental training on the philosophy of person-centered planning. The scale can also be completed by team members themselves.

How to evaluate and use the feedback: The results are shared with the planning team, and discussion focuses on strengths and weaknesses of the planning team interaction.

Planning Team Exercise 6: What Is Our Team Working Toward?

> **Purpose:** To refresh planning team member motivation and team processes after planning has been well underway. This exercise can increase group cohesion and provide a sense of common purpose among members. It can be especially helpful in refocusing group efforts during times of inaction or team conflict.

Information source: Eleven Principles of PICTURE

How to obtain the information: The worksheet is completed by team consensus during a meeting. The facilitator leads the exercise while members reach consensus about the status of each principle in relation to the team's current planning process.

How to evaluate and use the feedback: In discussing which options correspond most closely to the team's efforts in assisting the person with a disability, ideas about what the team could be working on or doing differently will occur. Variations of the exercise include 1) sorting and evaluating principles by status or 2) asking team members to select and discuss some principles to which the team conforms versus those that are not central to the planning process.

EXERCISES FOR THE MANAGEMENT TEAM

The organization must accommodate person-centered goals for person-centered planning to work in an agency. Recall that a person-centered team develops goals, plans for ways to accomplish those goals, receives feedback about its efforts, and then adjusts strategy. Likewise, the management team can plan for organizational changes that facilitate person-centered planning, receive feedback about their effectiveness, and revise strategy accordingly (see Figure 8 for an illustration of this process).

Examples of organizational strategies that promote person-centered planning might include training in implementing the approach, modes of transportation that favor individualization, policies and job descriptions that correspond to person-centered practices, board and committee membership by people with disabilities, newsletters and discussion groups that promote person-centered planning, and administration of staff surveys to assess agency performance.

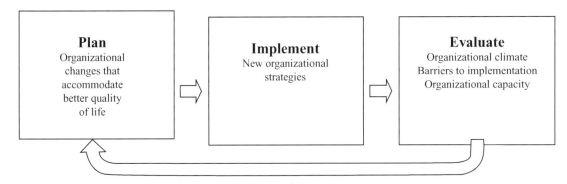

Figure 8.   Plan/implement/evaluate chart.

An organization that makes person-centered lifestyles possible must find ways to support individualized services. We suggest that the management team meet periodically to review what is and is not working to facilitate the goals established by the person-centered teams. Four exercises can be used to set management objectives for organizational change and to receive feedback on progress. Each exercise uses a different type of information that is derived from a different method. More sources will provide a clearer picture of the agency's capacity to support person-centered outcomes. The management team may already employ methods of evaluating organizational effectiveness; the critical factor here is the degree to which the methods are connected to the procedures,

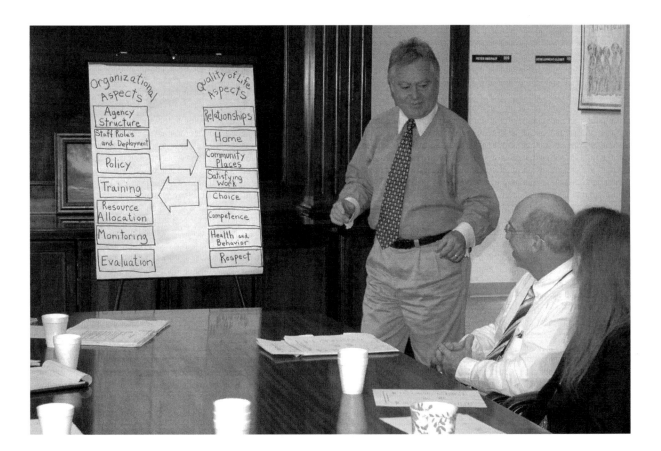

mechanisms, and cultural practices of the agency that directly impact the person's quality of life. The instruments and worksheets for the management exercises can be used to generate feedback to align management practices with the aspirations of the individuals being served by agency.

Suggested participants for the management self-evaluation exercises include key management personnel, such as the agency director, finance manager, clinical coordinator, personnel director, and other administrative employees. We also suggest participation by an individual with a disability, family member, and board member. The management self-evaluation meetings should occur on a regular basis, at least quarterly. We suggest a collaborative method, such as total quality management, as an organizing structure for the meetings, and we suggest flip charts for displaying and clarifying information during problem solving.

Management Exercise 1:
Creating a More Person-Centered Climate in Your Agency

> **Purpose:** Identify and alter staff attitudes.

Information source: Person-Centered Organizational Climate Survey

How to obtain the information: This survey can be administered to employees at all levels and functions. Confidentiality is crucial. The survey is not designed for use by individuals with disabilities.

How to evaluate the feedback: The answers to the 17 questions can be quantified, averaged, and analyzed by job category or function, or as an entire agency. Goals for improvement can be established, targeting areas of relative weakness. Ideally, the survey should be readministered to the same respondents. If job turnover is a problem, be sure to assess a sizable number of employees to ensure stability of results.

Management Exercise 2:
Removing Organizational Barriers to Person-Centered Outcomes

> **Purpose:** Identify and address organizational obstacles encountered by teams in helping individuals achieve their goals.

Information source: Barriers to Plan Implementation Form

How to obtain the information: This form should be completed by a member of the person-centered planning team, preferably the facilitator or his or her designee.

How to evaluate the feedback: Compile a list of obstacles and sort them by quality of life aspects. This is an efficient way to identify organizational impediments to the teams. Patterns will emerge that suggest areas of management intervention.

Management Exercise 3:
Organizational Processes that Facilitate Quality of Life

> **Purpose:** Ascertain the fit between organizational processes and person-centered goals, highlight organizational aspects that are misaligned, and suggest ways to improve the fit.

Information source: Relationship Between the Organization and Quality-of-Life Outcomes worksheet

How to obtain the information: Distribute this form at a management self-evaluation meeting. Participants are asked to consider each organizational aspect and whether it facilitates the outcomes listed on the right. The facilitator of the meeting then asks participants to consider each quality-of-life outcome, one at a time, and brainstorm changes in organizational aspects on the left that might foster the quality-of-life outcome.

How to evaluate the feedback: The ideas should be displayed on chart paper. The group will immediately identify some ideas as fitting and viable; the utility of others will be less clear. In a more elaborate version of this exercise, team members examine their suggestions for improvement by evaluating details of each aspect. For example, for Agency Structure, the organizational chart would be available; for Staff Roles and Deployment, selected job descriptions might be available; for Training, training programs or curricula could be available; and so forth.

Management Exercise 4:
Increasing Organizational Capacity for Person-Centered Outcomes

> **Purpose:** This exercise is intended to suggest specific ways an organization can improve its capacity to facilitate person-centered practices.

Information source: Person-Centered Organizational Capacity Indicators

How to obtain the information: Distribute this form at a management self-evaluation meeting. This is a group exercise in which the facilitator of the meeting reviews each capacity indicator, and participants discuss the relevance of the indicator to their agency or work group.

How to evaluate the feedback: Ideas are discussed for implementing or improving on existing indicators. Reviewing the indicators often leads to suggestions about modifying existing practices or developing new strategies not listed on the worksheet.

PART IV

Tools to Use with PICTURE: A Troubleshooter's Guide, Questionnaires, and Worksheets

The following section contains a troubleshooter's guide to using PICTURE and 10 evaluation tools used in PICTURE. The tools are used to evaluate the person's experiences, the planning team process, and the organizational support. Each assessment tool is linked to a planning exercise as described in Part III. Instructions for and use of the assessments are provided in the exercises and on the instruments themselves. See Table 4 for a summary of assessment instruments and corresponding exercises.

A TROUBLESHOOTER'S GUIDE: ISSUES OF PRINCIPLE

> **Problem:** Person-centered planning is misinterpreted as an impractical, dreamy endeavor that goes too far and provides unrealistic expectations to the person.

Try This: True, person-centered planners ask the person to dream big, but they do not offer the moon. The process seeks to tap into the person's capacities and then uses the skills of the team members to help him or her obtain a more rewarding lifestyle. Remind the detractor that many people with disabilities live isolated lives of undeveloped potential and are rarely given the chance to say how they would like to live their lives.

Table 4.   Summary of Assessment Instruments and Corresponding Exercises

Evaluation Tools	Exercises
The Person's Experiences	
Person-Centered Quality-of-Life Indicators	Taking a Look at Overall Quality of Life
Community Activities Checklist	Increasing Community Participation
Decision-Making and Satisfaction Interview	Keeping the Focus on the Person
Person-Centered Planning Team Process	
Assessment of Person-Centered Planning Facilitation Integrity	Conducting a Person-Centered Planning Meeting
Assessment of Person-Centered Planning Team Integrity	How Person-Centered Is Our Planning Team?
Eleven Principles of PICTURE Worksheet	What Is Our Team Working Toward?
Organizational Support	
Person-Centered Organizational Climate Survey	Creating a More Person-Centered Climate in Your Agency
Barriers to Plan Implementation Form	Removing Organizational Barriers to Person-Centered Outcomes
Relationship Between the Organization and Quality-of-Life Outcomes	Organizational Processes that Facilitate Quality of Life
Person-Centered Organizational Capacity Indicators	Increasing Organizational Capacity for Person-Centered Outcomes

---

Problem: The sentiment is expressed that people with intellectual disabilities do not have the cognitive capacity to make important decisions.

Try This: Of course a person with an intellectual disability does not have absolute dominion and authority in decision making. Making important choices entails negotiation, especially when health or safety is at stake (see Wehmeyer, 1998).

Problem: The sentiment is expressed that people with intellectual disabilities may be stressed or confused with too many decisions to make.

Try This: Remind the detractor that some people are not given the opportunity to decide what to eat, when to go to bed, or with whom to spend their time. Start with the smaller decisions first. It will not be difficult for the person with a disability to select preferred activities identified through the PICTURE process.

Problem: The sentiment is expressed that person-centered planning might work in other places but it cannot work here.

Try This: Suggest that person-centered planning is only as effective as the group members are able and willing to assist. Give examples of where person-centered planning has worked in rural as well as in urban environments. If needed, examples can be found in the Recommended Reading section of this manual.

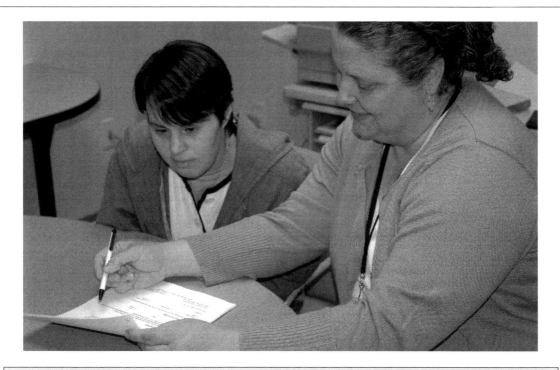

Problem: The opinion is offered that the community is not ready or prepared for a person who has considerable medical or behavioral problems and needs significant support.

Try This: Anyone can live in the community with the proper services and supports, although it can be difficult to arrange and maintain sufficient physical and behavioral health. Find out about ways that others have done this (see, e.g., Holburn & Vietze, 2002, in the Recommended Reading section). The transition to the community might be made easier if neighbors understand about disabilities.

Problem: The person with a disability is happy living in a congregate care environment. Does the person *have* to move into the community?

Try This: Not everyone wants to live in the community, but many people have not been given the choice to participate in community life. Honor the person's decision to live where he or she wants, especially if it is an informed decision based on knowledge and experience of community life.

Problem: Overzealous promotion of person-centered planning can give the impression that traditional services are ineffective and agency employees are doing a poor-quality job. Alienated employees will be reluctant to participate in the process.

Try This: Promoters and instructors of person-centered planning should emphasize that the approach requires the involvement of individuals who know and care about the person. But that is just the beginning. Participants with technical skills are essential. Person-centered planning will fail with individuals who need significant technical support if experts are not involved in the planning.

Problem: Overzealous promotion of person-centered planning has led to the impression that person-centered planning is a panacea.

Try This: Promoters and instructors of person-centered planning should emphasize that the method is not a cure-all; it is a gradual process that requires sustained effort. It does not supplant everything that preceded it—it builds on what the person has already learned.

Problem: The person with a disability has no clear preferences or interests outside of his or her current lifestyle. Decisions are always made *for* the person.

Try This: Introduce the person to various experiences from which he or she may learn about opportunities. Developing the eight life pictures outlined in this manual should give the team ideas about where to start.

Problem: The team is having second thoughts about pursuing a role for the person that sounded like a good idea at first but appears dangerous in some respects.

Try This: Imagine worst-case scenarios, and then imagine safeguards that might obviate the hazards. If the safeguards can feasibly be put into place, then the role might be achievable and safe. If not, then move on to secondary aspirations.

Problem: A person has an aspiration that is clearly unsafe, such as being a lifeguard even though he or she cannot swim or being a bus driver even though he or she cannot drive.

Try This: Introduce the person to roles related to the aspiration but scaled down to something more realistic. For example, the person who wants to be a lifeguard might be able to assist at a food stand or rental shop on the beach or perhaps gather recyclable and returnable materials on the beach. Swimming lessons would be another possibility to explore. The person who wants to be a bus driver might be satisfied as a courier who rides the bus.

Problem: An overprotective family member is the only team member who disagrees with a certain goal, believing that it cannot be accomplished or that it might put the person's safety in jeopardy.

Try This: Explain that plans often involve baby steps or small components to accomplish goals, and assure the family member that steps, plans, and goals can be adjusted. Encourage the parent to be become involved in or to observe the teaching, which could alleviate apprehension.

Problem: It is hard to know what the person really wants because his or her communication is poor.

Try This: Ensure that those who know the person best assist in speaking for the person. Some preferences can be validated empirically (see, e.g., Reid, Everson, & Green, 1999, for a systematic evaluation of preferences identified through person-centered planning).

Problem: The agency does not offer a service or program that addresses a goal important to the person.

Try This: This is a common conflict and requires creative thinking, problem solving, and knowledge about community resources. If the agency cannot develop the individualized service, then consider receiving services from an agency that offers a service related to the goal. The services may be offered by an agency unfamiliar with individuals with disabilities.

Problem: The plan for a better future is compromised because traditional funding is not sufficient to realize the plan.

Try This: Person-centered planners and funders work together to locate and merge available local, state, and federal resources. Invite managers with knowledge of fiscal matters to research solutions or assist with grant writing.

Problem: A family member who is important to the person has been disenfranchised by the agency and does not wish to participate in person-centered planning.

Try This: Encourage involvement by describing to the family member how person-centered planning is different than traditional approaches and that his or her involvement is valuable and important for the success of the planning. Encourage the person to invite the reluctant family member. Offer transportation assistance, if possible. A visit to the family member's home to explain the process could be the tipping point.

Problem: The person-centered planning team is stuck on an issue with no solution in sight.

Try This: Outside technical expertise is often needed when making significant changes in people's lives. Consider inviting an expert to the next meeting. It might be useful to establish an ad hoc subcommittee to investigate and learn more about the issue and devise a plan to break the roadblock.

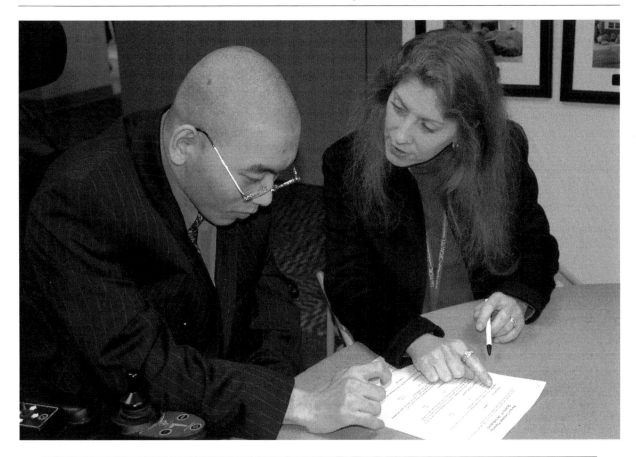

> **Problem:** The person-centered planning team appears to be floundering;
> there is disagreement about major goals and directions.

Try This: Periods of inaction and indecision can be a natural part of the process. It might be helpful to review the charts. Stay focused on what the person wants. Conduct the Eleven Principles of PICTURE: What Is Our Team Working Toward? exercise located in this section.

A TROUBLESHOOTER'S GUIDE: ORGANIZATIONAL ISSUES

> **Problem:** A power struggle exists in person-centered planning between
> professional opinion and family perspectives.

Try This: Explain that in person-centered planning, the traditional decision-making hierarchy gives way to a more egalitarian team process whereby all team members are considered equal. Remind the team that everyone's opinion is valuable to the process. However, PICTURE encourages professional support. Explain that team members need to keep an open mind, listen to others' perspectives, and work at solving problems. Ask, "What does the person with a disability want?" Keep the person at the center of the planning. It is likely that both parties are arguing for different means to the same end.

Problem: The agency is not sure how to begin to promote person-centered planning.

Try This: Consider revising the agency mission statement to reflect person-centered principles. This can be done as a group process to foster understanding and employee investment. Hold discussion groups among staff to talk about the principles of person-centered planning, how it might be implemented, and some of the problems and solutions that might be encountered in trying to implement it. Consider starting a few person-centered planning endeavors as demonstrations.

Problem: Managers enthusiastically promote person-centered planning, but employees are skeptical.

Try This: Accept dissenting perspectives and use them as a basis for frank discussion about the barriers and uncertainties that surface. Hold brainstorming sessions with staff about how to affect more inclusion, better relationships, and more choice making (see, e.g., Holburn & Vietze, 1999, in the Recommended Reading section).

Problem: Agency goals and practices do not coincide with person-centered values and approaches.

Try This: Acknowledge the divide between the concepts and goals of person-centered planning versus the agency's current capacity to implement it. Invite employees from all strata of the agency to participate in problem-solving sessions and work groups to consider reasonable adaptations within their own agency that could facilitate individualized services.

Problem: Person-centered planning is taking place very slowly in the agency; a relative few are involved in the process while others receive conventional service planning, which seems unfair.

Try This: Remind others that person-centered planning is done one person at a time, and ask, "Is it better to more fairly distribute a less desirable approach?" Explain that as person-centered planning is nurtured in the agency, the principles and practices spill over to some degree to individuals who are not part of a formal person-centered planning endeavor. Eventually, as the agency becomes more person-centered, more individualized planning and services will become available.

Problem: Person-centered planning has begun with all individuals with disabilities in the agency, but system resources are overwhelmed.

Try This: Focus on a smaller number of people for person-centered planning while working on system changes that will affect all individuals with disabilities.

Problem: The agency is promoting person-centered planning, but employee time is absorbed by regulatory compliance activities and paperwork.

Try This: Explore possibilities of other ways of deploying staff (some staff members prefer quality assurance activities). Flexible rules may be reinterpreted as fostering practices that contribute to more individualized lifestyles. Invite regulators and program auditors to open discussions about resolving potential regulatory impediments to honoring a person's interests and preferences.

Person-Centered Planning Quality-of-Life Indicators

Name of person: _____ Date: _____

Location/address: _____

Name of person completing this form: _____

This survey assesses eight aspects of a person's quality of life. Please read each question and check the box that represents the best answer. Please answer every question.

Home

1. Neighborhood

How many of the following characteristics describe the person's neighborhood? (a) safe, (b) clean, (c) convenient, (d) attractive:

☐ One ☐ Two ☐ Three ☐ All four ☐ None

2. Exterior physical qualities

How many of the following aspects describe the external physical qualities of the home? 1) attractive, 2) in good repair, 3) the size of the home blends into the neighborhood, 4) the architectural style of the home fits in well with the others:

☐ One ☐ Two ☐ Three ☐ All four ☐ None

3. Interior physical qualities

How many of the following aspects describe the interior of the home? (a) comfortable, relaxing atmosphere; (b) clean; (c) sufficient personal space and privacy; (d) good lighting, air quality, and room temperature:

☐ One ☐ Two ☐ Three ☐ All four ☐ None

4. Roommates/housemates

Generally speaking, the person and his or her housemates get along:

☐ Very well ☐ Well ☐ Fairly well ☐ Not so well ☐ Poorly

5. Staff

The person seems to be

☐ Well matched with all staff   ☐ Well matched with most staff

☐ Well matched with about half of the staff   ☐ Poorly matched with most staff

☐ Poorly matched with all staff

(continued)

6. Daily home routine

In an ideal daily routine, the person (a) learns functional skills (b) in an individualized, flexible routine (c) in which he or she is actively involved with others, and (d) has a good time doing it. How many of the previous elements are part of the person's daily routine?

☐ One ☐ Two ☐ Three ☐ All four ☐ None

Work, School, or Day Activity

7. Environment

Some important considerations of a work, school, or day activity environment include space, lighting, noise level, potential health hazards, other co-workers or classmates, and whether there is a friendly, supportive atmosphere. Considering these factors, how would you characterize the person's work, school, or day activity environment?

☐ Excellent ☐ Very good ☐ Good ☐ Fair ☐ Poor

8. Inclusion

During the course of the work, school, or day activity, the person spends time with co-workers and peers who do not have disabilities:

☐ Almost always ☐ Usually ☐ Sometimes ☐ Seldom ☐ Almost never

9. Responsibility

During the work, school, or day activity, the person does things by him- or herself in a way that increases his or her skills and competence:

☐ Almost always ☐ Usually ☐ Sometimes ☐ Seldom ☐ Almost never

10. Advancement

In the person's current work, school, or day activity, he or she will be promoted to job duties or educational activities of greater complexity, pay, or other benefit:

☐ Almost certainly ☐ Very likely ☐ Likely ☐ Somewhat likely ☐ Unlikely

11. Satisfaction

Overall, how satisfied is the person with the work, school, or day activity? (Where applicable, consider the duties, co-workers or classmates, setting, supervision, and pay and benefits.)

☐ Completely satisfied ☐ Highly satisfied ☐ Moderately satisfied

☐ Minimally satisfied ☐ Unsatisfied

Health

12. General health

The person's general health is:

☐ Excellent   ☐ Very good   ☐ Good   ☐ Fair   ☐ Poor

13. Personal health practices

Taken altogether, the person's health-related behaviors, routines, and practices are:

☐ Excellent for his or her health   ☐ Very good for his or her health

☐ Good for his or her health   ☐ Fair for his or her health

☐ Poor for his or her health

14. Health care

How would you describe the person's health care services, considering the need for medication, therapy, monitoring, equipment, and so forth?

☐ Excellent   ☐ Very good   ☐ Good   ☐ Fair   ☐ Poor

15. Emergency medical support

In case of a medical emergency, the person will have timely access to health care:

☐ Almost certainly   ☐ Very likely   ☐ Likely

☐ Somewhat likely   ☐ Unlikely

16. Emergency psychological support

In case of a psychological or behavioral emergency, the person will have timely access to people who will know how to assist:

☐ Almost certainly   ☐ Very likely   ☐ Likely

☐ Somewhat likely   ☐ Unlikely

Relationships

17. Friends

How many friends does the person have whom he or she is able to spend sufficient time with (not counting family)?

☐ A lot of friends   ☐ More than a few friends   ☐ A few friends

☐ One friend   ☐ No friends

18. Family members

Contact between the person and family members occurs approximately:

☐ Daily ☐ Weekly ☐ Monthly

☐ Semiannually ☐ Less than semiannually

19. Intimacy

If the person were interested in developing an intimate relationship with someone, would this be encouraged or supported?

☐ Definitely yes ☐ Probably yes ☐ Possibly

☐ Probably not ☐ Definitely not

20. Associations

How would you characterize the person's involvement in associations such as clubs, church, leagues, or other organized groups?

☐ Active participation on frequent basis   ☐ Active participation on occasional basis

☐ Passive participation on frequent basis   ☐ Passive participation on occasional basis

☐ No participation

21. Social network in community

In the community the person has:

☐ A rich network of friends and acquaintances   ☐ A sufficient number of friends and acquaintances

☐ A few friends and acquaintances and is actively developing more   ☐ No consistent contacts now, but is beginning to meet people

☐ No social contacts now, and there are no plans to develop any

Community Places

22. Community recreational locations

Approximately how often does the person go to places in the community for recreational purposes? Examples are ballpark, bowling alley, swimming pool, community center, church, clubs, theaters, museums.

☐ Daily ☐ Weekly ☐ Monthly

☐ Semiannually ☐ Less than semiannually

(continued)

23. Local neighborhood settings

Approximately how often does the person go to places in the local neighborhood? Examples are parks, schools, neighborhood walks, visiting others' homes, and so forth.

☐ Daily ☐ Weekly ☐ Monthly

☐ Semiannually ☐ Less than semiannually

24. Places to spend money

Approximately how often does the person go to business establishments in the community? Examples are restaurant, grocery store, coffee shop, department store, convenience store, delicatessen, barber shop, drug store, and bank.

☐ Daily ☐ Weekly ☐ Monthly

☐ Semiannually ☐ Less than semiannually

Preferences/Choices

25. Home

In decisions about the home, what impact do the person's desires, preferences, and interests have? Consider decisions about the location, space needs, furnishings, decor, bedroom arrangement, pets, and so forth.

☐ Very high impact ☐ High impact ☐ Some impact

☐ Low impact ☐ Very low impact

26. Work, school, or day activity

The person's desires, preferences, and interests are important considerations in deciding what the person does every day on the job, during school, or in the day activity:

☐ I agree strongly ☐ I agree ☐ I agree somewhat

☐ I disagree ☐ I disagree strongly

27. Food

The person makes choices about when to eat and what the meals consist of:

☐ Almost always ☐ Usually ☐ Sometimes

☐ Seldom ☐ Almost never

28. Appearance

The person makes decisions affecting his or her appearance, including choices about clothing, personal hygiene, hairstyle, facial hair, jewelry, and so forth:

☐ Almost always ☐ Usually ☐ Sometimes

☐ Seldom ☐ Almost never

29. Sleep and waking

The person decides when to go to bed, when to get up, and if/when to take naps:

☐ Almost always ☐ Usually ☐ Sometimes

☐ Seldom ☐ Almost never

30. Leisure activities

The person's preferences and interests determine what the person does in his or her spare time, including where to go, who to visit, what to watch on television, what music to listen to, and whether to decline to take part in a planned leisure activity:

☐ Almost always ☐ Usually ☐ Seldom

☐ Sometimes ☐ Almost never

31. New experiences

The person comes in contact with new and varied experiences that can become part of his or her repertoire of interests and preferences:

☐ Very frequently ☐ Frequently ☐ Once in a while

☐ Occasionally ☐ Almost never

32. Minor vices

The person can engage in minor vices such as smoking, drinking alcohol, overeating, drinking coffee with caffeine, and reading sexually explicit magazines:

☐ Any time he or she wishes ☐ Some things any time, other things with permission

☐ Occasionally with permission only ☐ Once in a while with permission only

☐ Almost never

Respect

33. Stigmatization

The person's environment and activities minimize the potential for stigmatizing the person. The person is not involved in conspicuous routines, schedules, or group activities with other people with disabilities. The home, workplace, or school and form of transportation do not call negative attention to the person:

☐ I agree strongly ☐ I agree ☐ I agree somewhat

☐ I disagree ☐ I disagree strongly

34. Personal appearance

The person's appearance promotes dignity and respect. He or she is well groomed and wears fashionable clothing that fits and is appropriate for the occasion:

☐ I agree strongly ☐ I agree ☐ I agree somewhat

☐ I disagree ☐ I disagree strongly

35. Contribution

The person assumes a valued social role. The person's work or day activity is an important part of a product or service or has other benefit to society; or if in school, the person's education is clearly preparing him or her for a valued social role:

☐ I agree strongly ☐ I agree ☐ I agree somewhat

☐ I disagree ☐ I disagree strongly

36. Public behavior

The person's behavior in public sets him or her apart from others and jeopardizes community acceptance:

☐ Never ☐ Rarely ☐ Once in a while

☐ Occasionally ☐ Frequently

37. Positive modeling

In the presence of others, family and staff communicate with the person in a manner that promotes a positive social image:

☐ I agree strongly ☐ I agree ☐ I agree somewhat

☐ I disagree ☐ I disagree strongly

Enhancing Competence

38. Effective teaching

The teaching strategies being used to improve personal care, communication, social interaction, and community living are known to be effective and are applied consistently:

☐ Almost always   ☐ Usually   ☐ Sometimes

☐ Seldom   ☐ Almost never

39. Skill relevance

How relevant are the skills that the person is currently learning to enhance his or her competence for living in the community, building relationships, and fostering vocational interests and skills?

☐ Completely relevant ☐ Highly relevant   ☐ Moderately relevant

☐ Minimally relevant ☐ Irrelevant

40. Control of lifestyle

The person is learning to exert greater control over the circumstances in her or his life that help achieve personal aspirations and goals:

☐ I agree strongly   ☐ I agree   ☐ I agree somewhat

☐ I disagree   ☐ I disagree strongly

Community Activities Checklist

Name of person: _____ Date: _____

Location/address: _____

Name of person completing this form: _____

Instructions:

In the "Visited" column, mark the community locations where the person went during the past 2 weeks (i.e., the 14 preceding days before the survey is completed). Using the next two columns, indicate if the person was accompanied by staff. Then, mark whether the person enjoyed the experience. If an activity can be categorized by more than one location, then choose the category that best describes the location. If the location is not listed in the checklist, then please mark "Other" and write in the location in the space provided.

Note: To qualify, an activity must take place in a community setting. A *community setting* is defined as a place where the majority of people present do not have developmental disabilities or where the principal purpose is something other than providing services and supports to people with developmental disabilities.

Visited	With staff	Without staff	Enjoyed?		Visited	With staff	Without staff	Enjoyed?	
Y N	O	O	Y N		Y N	O	O	Y N	
Y N	O	O	Y N	A friend's home	Y N	O	O	Y N	Parade
Y N	O	O	Y N	A family member's home	Y N	O	O	Y N	Party/picnic/barbecue
Y N	O	O	Y N	A friend's workplace	Y N	O	O	Y N	Pharmacy
Y N	O	O	Y N	A family member's workplace	Y N	O	O	Y N	Play/concert/performance
Y N	O	O	Y N	Airport, train station, or bus depot	Y N	O	O	Y N	Recreational/leisure class
Y N	O	O	Y N	Auto repair shop	Y N	O	O	Y N	Religious services/house of worship
Y N	O	O	Y N	Bank	Y N	O	O	Y N	Restaurant
Y N	O	O	Y N	Barber shop or hair salon	Y N	O	O	Y N	Retail store
Y N	O	O	Y N	Dry cleaners or launderers	Y N	O	O	Y N	Sightseeing
Y N	O	O	Y N	Club meeting	Y N	O	O	Y N	Scheduled outing
Y N	O	O	Y N	Community park	Y N	O	O	Y N	Sport or athletic activity (as participant)
Y N	O	O	Y N	Convenience store	Y N	O	O	Y N	Supermarket
Y N	O	O	Y N	Doctor's office (e.g., general medical practice)	Y N	O	O	Y N	Video store
Y N	O	O	Y N	Educational class	Y N	O	O	Y N	Volunteer work

(continued)

Visited	With staff	Without staff	Enjoyed?		Visited	With staff	Without staff	Enjoyed?	
Y N	O	O	Y N		Y N	O	O	Y N	
Y N	O	O	Y N	Exhibit/show	Y N	O	O	Y N	Worksite
Y N	O	O	Y N	Fair/festival	Y N	O	O	Y N	Zoo/aquarium/nature park
Y N	O	O	Y N	Fast-food restaurant					Other (please list below)
Y N	O	O	Y N	Game room/arcade/ recreational facility	Y N	O	O	Y N	
Y N	O	O	Y N	Gymnasium/exercise facility	Y N	O	O	Y N	
Y N	O	O	Y N	Hobby shop	Y N	O	O	Y N	
Y N	O	O	Y N	Laundromat	Y N	O	O	Y N	
Y N	O	O	Y N	Library	Y N	O	O	Y N	
Y N	O	O	Y N	Live sports event (as spectator)	Y N	O	O	Y N	
Y N	O	O	Y N	Mall	Y N	O	O	Y N	
Y N	O	O	Y N	Movie/theater	Y N	O	O	Y N	
Y N	O	O	Y N	Museum	Y N	O	O	Y N	
Y N	O	O	Y N	Outdoor activity (e.g., walks, park, beach)	Y N	O	O	Y N	

Decision-Making and Satisfaction Interview

Name of person: _____ Date: _____

Location/address: _____

Name of parent or advocate: _____

Name of interviewer: _____

Instructions:
This interview may be conducted with the individual with a disability, his or her parents, or an advocate, as appropriate. The perspective that should be taken in answering the questions is that of the individual, regardless of who responds to the questions. Reword the question if the respondent appears to be unsure of its meaning. Prompt for additional information to clarify ambiguous or incomplete answers.

Develop Rapport

First, engage the individual in a warm-up discussion about the person-centered planning with which (name of facilitator) has been helping him or her. Inform the person that you want to ask some questions about the person-centered planning and how happy he or she is (interviewer can elaborate).

Planning Process

1. Do you think that person-centered planning has changed your life very much? (If the person does not understand the question, then reword by referring to his or her involvement or planning with [name of facilitator]).

2. If "yes," then ask the person to tell you how.

3. What do you like best about the person-centered planning meetings? (Or, can you tell me some good things about the person-centered planning meetings?)

4. Can you think of ways your person-centered planning meetings could be better?

5. If "yes," then ask the person to tell you how.

6. Do people listen to what you say during the person-centered planning meetings?

7. Do you get to make important decisions about your life?

8. If "yes," then ask the person to give you an example.

9. Would you like to make more decisions about your life? (Or, do you want people to listen more to what you have to say?)

10. If "yes," then ask the person what other decisions he or she would like to make.

General Satisfaction

For this part, ask the respondent if he or she is satisfied with the following life aspects and if he or she wants assistance in any of these areas. If necessary, reword the life aspect for clarity.

Are you satisfied with this area of your life? (Write yes or no)	Do you want help in this area? (Write yes or no)
_____ Relationships	_____ Relationships
_____ Home life	_____ Home life
_____ Work, school, or day activity	_____ Work, school, or day activity
_____ Community places	_____ Community places
_____ Community competence	_____ Community competence
_____ Respect	_____ Respect
_____ Physical and behavioral health	_____ Physical and behavioral health
_____ Preferences and choices	_____ Preferences and choices

How much direct input was given by the person during the interview?

1. All questions were answered by the person (i.e., no input from others was needed).

2. Most questions were answered by the person (i.e., a little input from others was needed).

3. A few questions were answered by the person (i.e., a lot of input from others was needed).

4. No questions were answered by the person (i.e., all input was from others).

Information from the Assessment of Person-Centered Planning Facilitation Integrity is used to determine facilitator adherence to the **22 person-centered planning meeting components** listed. The results can be shared with the facilitator or the entire team to provide feedback and maintain the quality of the person-centered planning process. It may also be used as a research tool to report on the degree of fidelity to the planning process as defined by the items and criteria described.

The assessment should be filled out immediately after the meeting, preferably by an independent observer (i.e., someone who is not on the planning team), but if this is not possible or if the person is not comfortable with an independent observer attending the meeting, then a member of the planning team may serve as respondent.

The following criteria will help determine whether to specify *Y* (yes), *N* (no), or *NA* (not appropriate) in response to each question.

1. Date and time of meeting was convenient for the person.

The date and time should be arranged for convenience of the person. The evaluator should inquire as to whether these factors were taken into consideration when arranging the meeting. Indicate *NA* if it is not possible for the person to attend.

2. Meeting location was adequate.

The meeting should take place in a location with enough space. Attendees should be able to sit comfortably without feeling cramped. The walls should accommodate wall charts. The atmosphere should be relaxed with minimal distractions or disruptions such as staff responding to other duties, excessive noise, or inadequate temperature or lighting. The space should be private enough for the person and team members to feel comfortable in speaking freely about personal issues.

3. Seating arrangement facilitated discussion.

Participants should be able to see and hear each other easily. Wall charts should be visible. People who are not agency employees (e.g., the person, family members, friends) should sit up front or close to the facilitator, where they are more likely to participate. They should not be seated in a way that deters their interaction (not in back of others or away from group).

4. Refreshments were available.

Food and drink enhance the social process. At least a beverage should be available.

5. Charting materials (e.g., flip charts, markers) were present at meeting.

Charting can improve communication and problem solving among team members by providing visible information of the meeting proceedings. These charts can be referred to throughout the meeting for expansion or clarification of issues. The charts can also be displayed at later meetings. Charting is an inherent aspect of the person-centered planning process and especially important in the early stages of the planning. Charting materials should be sufficient, available, and located in the planning room.

6. **Attempts were made to get relevant people at the meeting, including timely notification and, if feasible, transportation assistance.**

The evaluator may have to unobtrusively inquire about attempts to get key people to attend the meeting. The facilitator or designee should invite people who know the person well, who can contribute to the planning process, and who are willing to help toward the pursuit of a better life for the person. Such people include, but are not limited to, the person with a disability, family members, friends, and pertinent staff members. It is not a clinical meeting. If all attendees are human services workers, then indicate *N*. Unless impossible or contraindicated, the person should be at the meeting and should feel comfortable with attendees.

7. **At the outset of the meeting, the facilitator stated the purpose of the meeting.**

At the beginning of each meeting, the facilitator should state briefly why the group is meeting and provide a general statement of what the group will be doing. Even at subsequent meetings after the process has been well established, the facilitator should summarize the purpose of that particular meeting and give an idea of the work ahead for the participants.

8. **Team progress was reviewed early in the meeting, including status of pending action steps.**

Early on, the facilitator should review the successes and developments of the prior meeting(s). The facilitator should review each pending strategy and action step and ask relevant participants to report on what they said they would do.

9. **The facilitator asked probing, open-ended questions to evoke detail about the person and issues related to him or her.**

The facilitator must get group members talking to extract important and often overlooked information about the life of the person. Effective facilitators use a variety of questioning styles. For example, instead of asking, "Does she ever go to the store?" the facilitator might ask, "Where does she go in the community?" Likewise, instead of asking, "Does she enjoy swimming?" the facilitator might ask, "What does she like to do?" When answers such as "yes" or "no" do not convey enough information, the facilitator should respond by asking a follow-up question such as, "Can you tell us a little more about that?"

10. **The facilitator kept the discussion centered on the interests and desires of the person.**

The interests and wishes of the person with a disability must remain the central point of focus. When the group digresses, the facilitator should redirect the discussion toward the person. If there is confusion about what the group should be working toward, whether it is a small issue (e.g., the color of a new coat) or a large issue (e.g., the type of neighborhood that would be best to move into), then the facilitator should keep the group focused on what the person wants. Although the person's interests are vital, sometimes the facilitator must get the group to make a decision that balances health and safety with the person's aspirations.

11. **The facilitator was oriented more toward building capacity than toward correcting deficiencies.**

The facilitator should solicit information about the person's strengths, abilities, and interests and should build on this information to develop ideas for a better quality of life. Not a great deal of time should be spent discussing clinical issues or the person's shortcomings that appear to be obstacles to achievement. The facilitator's role is not to identify deficiencies for professional remediation or amelioration; rather, he or she should identify and build on the person's current skills and capacities that will facilitate social inclusion. For example, a discussion might focus on what skills must be improved for enhancing community inclusion, making friends, or getting a job. The facilitator should guide the team toward positive approaches to solve problems that arise.

12. **Throughout the meeting, the facilitator sought clarification of vague information and cloudy issues.**

Sometimes team members do not ask for clarification when participants use terms or acronyms that are unclear, have multiple meanings, or are stated in a glib manner. It is the responsibility of the facilitator to seek clarification of such information so that everyone understands what was expressed. Likewise, when there are many aspects or dimensions to an issue or problem, the facilitator should restate these aspects and present them in a way that helps the team solve the problem.

13. **The facilitator conveyed an optimistic attitude.**

The facilitator should show enthusiasm in focusing on positive attributes of the person and in helping the group create a picture of a better quality of life for the person. The facilitator should guide the group in a manner that engenders excitement about the possibilities and inspires confidence in making the picture become a reality. When the challenges appear insurmountable or when there are droughts of inaction, the facilitator keeps confidence alive by reminding members of their accomplishments so far and the importance of their mission.

14. **The facilitator encouraged creative solutions during problem solving.**

The facilitator communicates a can-do attitude about helping the person accomplish goals. Members are encouraged to think outside the box when listening to the views of others and to be open to their ideas. Participants are encouraged to "think big" or "dream big" and to imagine innovative ways to make the dream come true. In the absence of criticism, members are more likely to brainstorm possible solutions and generate different ways of solving problems.

15. **If present system constraints prevented achievement of the person's wish(es), then alternative ways of achievement were discussed.**

When system policies, structure, or lack of resources prevent achievement of a person-centered goal, the facilitator should encourage creative problem solving, rather than giving up the struggle to reach the goal. For example, the team might discuss ways of getting outside resources to achieve a goal or discuss possibilities of different internal system policies, structure, and so forth that would accommodate the person. If there is no discussion of system constraint impeding solutions, specify *NA.*

16. **The facilitator obtained consensus in problem solving.**

The facilitator should seek solutions by getting everyone involved and invested in the process. The solution should reflect members' shared ideas, including those of the person with a disability. The goal for which the solution is sought is reviewed, and differences in ideas are clarified and discussed. When there is not full agreement, solutions are weighed and one is selected that is acceptable to most members of the group.

17. The facilitator gave positive feedback to participants when they shared information.

The facilitator should respond positively (e.g., smiling, nodding, saying encouraging words) when team members share information that contributes to the person-centered process. The absence of such feedback will limit member input. If you believe that the facilitator did not sufficiently reward participants in this manner, then indicate *N*.

18. If charting was used, it conveyed information in a way that helped team members develop a common understanding of the person.

The charts should be hung on the wall or displayed in a way that can be easily seen by all. Text and graphic information should be presented in a clear and understandable manner. The information on the charts should reflect the contributions of participants, including the person. The information should convey a greater understanding of the person's history, interests, goals, and feelings. The charts should be summarized occasionally during the meeting.

19. Strategies and responsibilities for follow-up were made clear.

When a team member makes a commitment to take action related to the plan, the facilitator should restate or clarify the strategy, document the action to be taken, and identify the time frame for achievement of the action.

20. All participants gave input during the meeting.

The facilitator should be sure that all team members express themselves during the meeting. To ensure such participation, the facilitator might ask each person to give their opinion on a particular issue or give their impression of the meeting before it concludes. Specify *Y* if the person cannot communicate clearly but others who are knowledgeable about the person spoke on his or her behalf. Specify *N* if the person is able to communicate but does not give input at the meeting.

21. The plan of action was summarized at the end of the meeting.

As the meeting is concluding, the facilitator should review the action steps. Preferably using the charts as a reference, he or she should remind team members of their commitments by restating each strategy, the person responsible for carrying it out, and the time frame for accomplishment.

22. A record of proceedings of the meeting information was kept.

Some form of written documentation, such as wall charts or notes, should occur as the meeting proceeds. The written record is used to maintain group cohesion, facilitate follow up, and enhance problem solving.

Assessment of Person-Centered Planning Facilitation Integrity

Name of person: _____ Date: _____

Name of facilitator: _____

Location/address: _____

Number of people at meeting: _____

Person at meeting? Yes _____ No _____

Place a *Y* (yes), *N* (no), or *NA* (not appropriate) before each question. See instructions and assessment criteria preceeding this form.

Arranging the Meeting

_____ 1. Date and time of meeting was convenient for the person.

_____ 2. Meeting location was adequate.

_____ 3. Seating arrangement facilitated discussion.

_____ 4. Refreshments were available.

_____ 5. Charting materials (e.g., flip charts, markers) were present at meeting.

_____ 6. Attempts were made to get relevant people at meeting, including timely notification and, if feasible, transportation.

Facilitating the Meeting

_____ 7. At the outset of the meeting, the facilitator stated the purpose of the meeting.

_____ 8. Team progress was reviewed early in the meeting, including status of pending action steps.

_____ 9. The facilitator asked probing, open-ended questions to evoke detail about the person and issues related to him or her.

_____ 10. The facilitator kept discussion centered on the interests and desires of the person.

_____ 11. The facilitator was oriented more toward building the individual's capacity than correcting his or her deficiencies.

_____ 12. Throughout the meeting, the facilitator sought clarification of vague information and cloudy issues.

_____ 13. The facilitator conveyed an optimistic attitude.

_____ 14. The facilitator encouraged creative solutions during problem solving.

_____ 15. If present system constraints prevented achievement of the person's wish(es), then alternative ways of achievement were discussed.

_____ 16. The facilitator obtained consensus in problem solving.

_____ 17. The facilitator gave positive feedback to participants when they shared information.

_____ 18. If charting was used, it conveyed information in a way that helped team members develop a common understanding of the person.

_____ 19. Strategies and responsibilities for follow-up were made clear.

_____ 20. All participants gave input during the meeting.

_____ 21. The plan of action was summarized at the end of the meeting.

_____ 22. A recording of proceedings was kept.

Notes:

Instructions and Assessment Criteria for Assessment of Person-Centered Planning Team Integrity

Information from the Assessment of Person-Centered Planning Team Integrity is used to determine adherence to **12 indicators of team member interaction** at a person-centered planning meeting. The results can be shared with team members to provide feedback to them and maintain the quality of the person-centered planning process. It may also be used as a research tool to report on the degree of fidelity to the planning process as defined by the items and criteria that follow.

The assessment should be filled out immediately after the meeting, preferably by an independent observer (someone who is not on the planning team), but if this is not possible or if the person is not comfortable with an independent observer attending the meeting, then a member of the planning team may serve as respondent.

The following criteria will help determine whether to specify *Y* (yes), *N* (no), or *NA* (not appropriate) in response to each question.

1. Used everyday language during the meeting (i.e., avoided professional jargon)

Team members speak as if they were at home or with friends. They avoid using professional terms or jargon when they talk during the meeting.

2. Viewed problems as opportunities for lifestyle improvements

Team members take advantage of difficulties that come up during the meeting and turn the problems into opportunities for change. If no problems emerge, then indicate *NA*.

3. Suggested solutions to problems

When problems emerge, the team members are active in making suggestions for solutions. This means that they are interested in solving the problem and instrumental in getting others to work on solutions as well. If no problems emerge, then indicate *NA*.

4. Were respectful of the person

Team members include the person in the discussion, ask him or her for suggestions, or offer alternatives and look for agreement. The team members also show respect in addressing the person and make eye contact. When talking about the person, the team members refrain from talking as if the person is not present. If the person is an adult, team members refrain from talking with the person or about the person as if he or she is a child. Indicate *NA* if person is not present.

5. Listened attentively to other team members

Team members use active listening techniques when other members are talking. They observe the speakers when they speak and wait until a speaker is finished talking before offering an opinion, feedback, or their own suggestions. They pay attention to each other and do not engage in other activities during the meeting, such as knitting or looking at their personal digital assistants, and they do not conduct other business during the meeting. When members participate in the discussion, they comment on what the previous speaker says rather than speaking in non sequitors.

6. Considered others' opinions

Members of the team think about what others members say during the meeting. They react to other team members' opinions or statements by using phrases such as "I agree" or "I disagree" and offer further explanation for their response.

7. Were not hindered in problem solving by an absence of important team members

If a team member who plays an important role is not present, other team members still contribute and function as a team. Problems are discussed and solutions are considered.

8. Promoted decision making by the person

Team members encourage the person to give his or her opinion about issues. If the person is reluctant to participate, then team members try to evoke participation. If the person does not understand an issue, then team members try to explain it to the person so he or she can understand it. Indicate *NA* if the person is not present.

9. Honored the person's preferences and choices

Team members listen to the person when he or she expresses a preference or choice. Members thoughtfully consider the idea, rather than dismissing it outright or ignoring it if it sounds unreasonable. They respond favorably and positively to the idea(s), at least initially, and attempt to negotiate alternatives if the expressed choice is a clear threat to health or safety.

10. Kept discussion centered on the person rather than each other or the agency

The discussion is principally focused on the person. The team is not diverted by tangential comments made by other team members. If the conversation begins to drift off topic, then team members guide the conversation back to the person and the person-centered process.

11. Were not negative in their expectations for the person

Team members maintain a positive attitude about the aspirations of the person. The overall outlook is that the person can be successful in his or her pursuits, rather than how difficult it would be for the person to achieve his or her goals.

12. Followed through with commitments made in the previous meeting

Team members carry out activities or plans that they committed to during the last meeting, as evidenced by discussion about the follow-up.

Assessment of Person-Centered Planning Team Integrity

Name of person: _____ Date: _____

Name of facilitator: _____

Location/address: _____

Was the person at the meeting? Yes _____ No _____

Number of people at meeting (not counting independent observer): _____

Instructions:

The items reflect team member interaction during a person-centered planning meeting. Estimate the degree to which you observed that the following indicators occurred during the meeting. (Please complete this survey immediately after the meeting.)

Indicators	No team members	Some team members	Most team members	All team members	NA
1. Used everyday language during meeting (i.e., avoided professional jargon)					
2. Viewed problems as opportunities for lifestyle improvements					
3. Suggested solutions to problems					
4. Were respectful of the person					
5. Listened attentively to other team members					
6. Considered others' opinions					
7. Were not hindered in problem solving by an absence of important team members					
8. Promoted decision making by the person					
9. Honored the person's preferences and choices					

Indicators	No team members	Some team members	Most team members	All team members	NA
10. Kept discussion centered on the person rather than each other or the agency					
11. Were not negative in their expectations for the person					
12. Followed through with previous meeting commitments					

Eleven Principles of PICTURE: What Is Our Team Working Toward?

Team members: _____ Date: _____

Facilitator: _____

Instructions: This survey should be completed by person-centered planning team members in group fashion. The facilitator leads the exercise while members reach consensus about the status of each principle in relation to the team's current planning process. Members determine which of the three options corresponds most closely to the team's efforts in assisting the person with a disability and a member or facilitator will write the appropriate letter in the corresponding space.

A   Our team is trying to do this

B   Our team has considered this but is not actively pursuing this

C   Our team has not considered this

_____   **People with disabilities should live like the rest of us.** PICTURE seeks to remove the stigma and get the person involved with the rest of the main culture, not trapped in a world consisting only of services.

_____   **Individualization is important.** PICTURE seeks to individualize routines and schedules in ways that promote personal decision making, expand the person's experiences, and develop his or her capacities.

_____   **The organization must be responsive.** PICTURE attempts to influence the organization to alter its planning, structure, policies, deployment of staff, allocation of resources, and forms of evaluation to promote person-centered supports and services.

_____   **Workers must be helpers.** PICTURE seeks to empower the employee to work more constructively and creatively, thus making the relationship more satisfying to the person with the disability and to the employee.

_____   **Members of the community must get involved.** PICTURE facilitates the development of community services and supports for people with disabilities so they can return to their communities. If the person already resides in the community, then the planning team seeks to improve the level of preferred community participation.

_____   **Real friendships are in the community.** Prerequisite to the development of real friendships, people with disabilities must be exposed to the community, and community members must have contact with people with disabilities.

_____   **Bring back the family.** PICTURE seeks to give power back to relatives and reunite families who have been disenfranchised and discouraged from maintaining regular contact with their loved one.

_____   **Start where you are; use what you have.** The PICTURE method does not abandon professional services and system components that are consistent with the person-centered approach—it needs them.

_____ **Team members take personal responsibility.** Many person-centered goals are achieved because team members take it on themselves to get the job done.

_____ **See the whole person.** PICTURE asks participants not to overfocus on any one aspect of the person. Seeing how one's history, abilities, and aspirations converge to form a picture of a better life requires consideration of many aspects of the person's life, or seeing the person as a whole.

_____ **Natural engagement is promoted.** PICTURE seeks to establish a more interesting and productive pattern of activities. The stimulation of preferred opportunities produces a natural engagement in the activities.

Person-Centered Organizational Climate Survey

Job title: _____ Date: _____

Instructions: This survey is designed to determine the extent to which the atmosphere in your agency is person centered. You may be asked to complete this survey again at a later date. *All answers will be kept strictly confidential. Do not include your name on this survey.*

For each item, check the box that indicates how you feel about the statement.

Indicator	Disagree	Disagree somewhat	Agree somewhat	Agree
1. My agency encourages me to be creative in finding ways to help people with disabilities achieve their personal goals.				
2. Staff talk with the individual's family members on a regular basis about opportunities for the individual to be involved in their local community.				
3. My agency helps people with disabilities pursue their interests, even if my agency does not offer those interests as part of their program.				
4. My agency empowers staff to find solutions to problems that interfere with community inclusion.				
5. My agency encourages people to ask for what they want to advocate for themselves.				
6. Agency management takes risks to help individuals get what they want.				
7. My agency encourages staff to help people build on what they are good at.				
8. My agency is willing to change its goals and procedures to help people with disabilities pursue their interests.				
9. People served by my agency are achieving their dreams and ambitions.				
10. My agency has clearly explained my role in helping people with disabilities have more choice in how they live their lives.				

Indicator	Disagree	Disagree somewhat	Agree somewhat	Agree
11. Management regularly asks staff about what is working and what is not working, with an emphasis on the aspirations of each person.				
12. People served by my agency tend to participate in community activities alone or with one or two other people, rather than in larger groups.				
13. My agency encourages me to honor people's choices and preferences.				
14. My agency has given me the training I need to help people be more included in their communities.				
15. My agency has given me the training I need to help people develop better relationships.				
16. My agency has given me the training I need to help people be more independent in their decision making.				
17. People with disabilities travel to community activities alone or with one or two other people, rather than in larger groups.				

Person-Centered Planning Made Easy: The PICTURE Method
By Steve Holburn, Anne Gordon, & Peter M. Vietze

Barriers to Plan Implementation Form

Name of person: _____ Date: _____

Name of facilitator: _____

Instructions: This form provides feedback to the management team about organizational obstacles to the outcomes the planning team is trying to achieve for the person with a disability. It should be completed by the facilitator or designee as follows: 1) state the goal, 2) indicate the quality of life aspect from the box, and 3) describe the obstacle in specific terms. Only describe obstacles that you feel are organizational barriers, such as policy, training, resources, staffing, and transportation.

QUALITY-OF-LIFE ASPECTS			
Relationship	Community places	Choice	Health and behavior
Home	Work, day, school	Competence	Respect

Goal 1

1. What goal is your team trying to achieve? _____

_____

2. What quality-of-life aspect does it reflect from the box? _____

_____

3. Describe the obstacles to this goal _____

_____

Goal 2

1. What goal is your team trying to achieve? _____

_____

2. What quality-of-life aspect does it reflect from the box? _____

_____

3. Describe the obstacles to this goal _____

_____

(continued)

Goal 3

1. What goal is your team trying to achieve? _____

_____

2. What quality-of-life aspect does it reflect from the box? _____

_____

3. Describe the obstacles to this goal _____

_____

Goal 4

1. What goal is your team trying to achieve? _____

_____

2. What quality-of-life aspect does it reflect from the box? _____

_____

3. Describe the obstacles to this goal _____

_____

Goal 5

1. What goal is your team trying to achieve? _____

_____

2. What quality-of-life aspect does it reflect from the box? _____

_____

3. Describe the obstacles to this goal _____

_____

The Relationship Between the Organization and Quality-of-Life Outcomes: Organizational Processes that Facilitate Quality of Life

This agency self-evaluation worksheet is designed to 1) assess the degree to which the organization is supporting person-centered aspirations, 2) identify aspects of the agency that are misaligned with those aspirations, and 3) serve as the basis for discussion about how to modify misaligned aspects.

Instructions: Distribute this worksheet at an agency management meeting, and explain the purpose as described above. Participants consider the degree to which organizational aspects on the left facilitate quality-of-life outcomes on the right. Each quality-of-life outcome is measured against each organizational aspect for degree of "fit." For example, beginning with *Relationships*, participants discuss how the *Relationships* aspect of quality of life is promoted or facilitated by the agency's *Structure, Staff roles and deployment, Policy, Training*, and so forth. Continue comparing each quality-of-life aspect with each organizational aspect.

As this exercise proceeds, patterns or rankings of organizational and quality-of-life aspects will begin to emerge that identify organizational aspects that are most and least supportive of the quality-of-life aspects. Discussion about how to modify misaligned organizational aspects and strengthen aligned aspects may proceed as individual comparisons are considered or after all comparisons have been made.

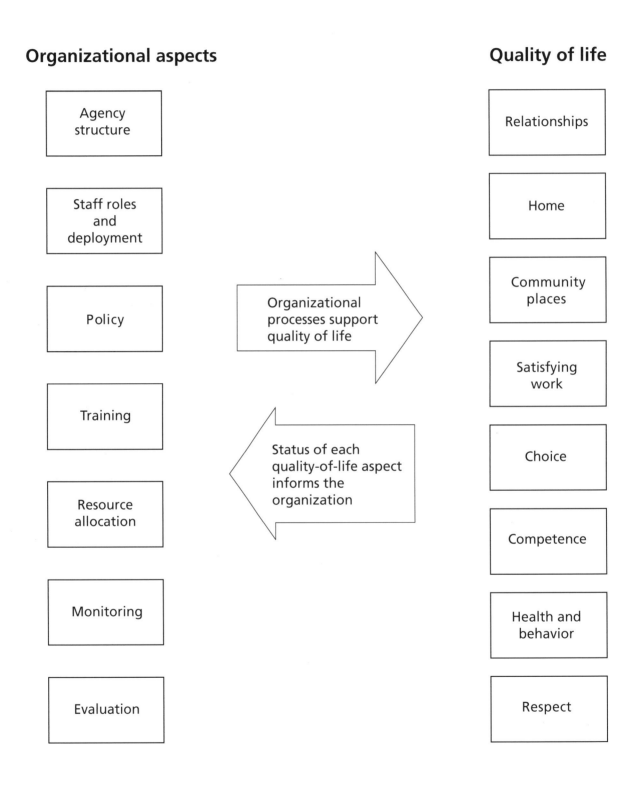

Organizational aspects

| Agency structure |
| Staff roles and deployment |
| Policy |
| Training |
| Resource allocation |
| Monitoring |
| Evaluation |

Organizational processes support quality of life →

← Status of each quality-of-life aspect informs the organization

Quality of life

| Relationships |
| Home |
| Community places |
| Satisfying work |
| Choice |
| Competence |
| Health and behavior |
| Respect |

Person-Centered Organizational Capacity Indicators: Increasing Organizational Capacity for Person-Centered Outcomes

Instructions:

This survey should be completed by management team members. Indicate whether the following are evident in your agency by writing *Y* (yes), *N* (no), or *NA* (not applicable) for each of the following.

_____ 1. Staff receive training in person-centered philosophy and practices.

_____ 2. Opportunities exist for making the transition to more individualized and inclusive school, work, or other day options or to smaller, more independent living arrangements.

_____ 3. People with disabilities have control or direct involvement in choices of supports and services.

_____ 4. People with disabilities have control or direct involvement in spending decisions.

_____ 5. Board membership includes individuals with disabilities.

_____ 6. Committee membership includes individuals with disabilities (one or more committees).

_____ 7. The agency recognizes individuals and teams that promote best practices in community inclusion, self-determination, and relationship building.

_____ 8. The agency has flexible funding mechanisms and opportunities.

_____ 9. There is a mission statement that references person-centered values and goals.

_____ 10. Management communicates with people with disabilities and staff to find out what is working and what is not working, with an emphasis on individuals' aspirations.

_____ 11. The agency collaborates with community resources in ways that promote inclusion.

_____ 12. The organization employs measures that assess quality of life to improve services.

_____ 13. The organization employs measures that assess satisfaction by people with disabilities to improve services.

_____ 14. Staff surveys assess how staff feel about their jobs.

_____ 15. The management team systematically evaluates its own capacity to provide individualized services and supports.

_____ 16. The organization promotes person-centered philosophy by disseminating information about person-centered principles (e.g., newsletters, bulletin boards, published literature).

_____ 17. The agency sponsors forums (e.g., conferences, meetings, discussion groups) that promote person-centered practices.

_____ 18. Job descriptions reflect a person-centered focus or they are being redesigned with that focus.

Recommended Reading

Holburn, S. (1997). A renaissance in residential behavior analysis? A historical perspective and a better way to help people with challenging behavior. *The Behavior Analyst, 20,* 61–85.

Holburn, S. (2002). How science can evaluate and enhance person-centered planning. *Research and Practice for Persons with Severe Disabilities, 27,* 250–260.

Holburn, S., & Jacobson, J.W. (2004). Implementing and researching person-centered planning. In L. Williams (Ed.), *Developmental disabilities: Advances in scientific understanding, clinical treatments, and community integration* (pp. 315–330). Reno, NV: Context Press.

Holburn, S., Jacobson, J.W., Schwartz, A., Flori, M., & Vietze, P. (2004). The Willowbrook futures project: A longitudinal analysis of person-centered planning. *American Journal on Mental Retardation, 109,* 63–76.

Holburn, C.S., & Pfadt, A. (1998). Clinicians on person-centered planning teams: New roles, fidelity of planning, and outcome assessment. *Mental Health Aspects of Developmental Disabilities, 1,* 82–86.

Holburn, C.S., & Vietze, P. (1999). Acknowledging barriers in adopting person-centered planning. *Mental Retardation, 37,* 117–124.

Holburn, S., & Vietze, P. (Eds.). (2002). *Person-centered planning: Research, practice, and future directions.* Baltimore: Paul H. Brookes Publishing Co.

Kincaid, D. (1996). Person-centered planning. In L.K. Koegel, R.L. Koegel, & G. Dunlap (Eds.), *Positive behavioral support: Including people with difficult behavior in the community* (pp. 439–465). Baltimore: Paul H. Brookes Publishing Co.

Mount, B. (1994). Benefits and limitations of personal futures planning. In V.J. Bradley, J.W. Ashbaugh, & B.C. Blaney (Eds.), *Creating individual supports for people with developmental disabilities: A mandate for change at many levels* (pp. 97–108). Baltimore: Paul H. Brookes Publishing Co.

O'Brien, J. (1987). A guide to life-style planning: Using the Activities Catalogue to integrate services and natural support systems. In G.T. Bellamy & B. Wilcox (Eds.), *A comprehensive guide to the Activities Catalogue: An alternative curriculum for youth and adults with severe disabilities* (pp. 175–189). Baltimore: Paul H. Brookes Publishing Co.

O'Brien, J.O. (2006). *Reflecting on social roles: Identifying opportunities to support personal freedom and social integration.* Version 1. Atlanta, GA: Responsive System Associates.

O'Brien, J., & Mount, B. (1991). Telling new stories: The search for capacity among people with severe handicaps. In L.H. Meyer, C.A. Peck, & L. Brown (Eds.), *Critical issues in the lives of people with severe disabilities* (pp. 89–92). Baltimore: Paul H. Brookes Publishing Co.

O'Brien, J., & O'Brien, C.L. (2002). (Eds.) *Implementing person-centered planning: Voices of experience.* Toronto: Inclusion Press.

Risley, T. (1996). Get a life! Positive behavioral intervention for challenging behavior through life arrangement and life coaching. In L.K. Koegel, R.L. Koegel, & G. Dunlap (Eds.), *Positive behavioral support: Including people with difficult behavior in the community* (pp. 425–437). Baltimore: Paul H. Brookes Publishing Co.

Sanderson, H., Kennedy, J., & Ritchie, P. (2003). *People, plans, and possibilities: Exploring person-centered planning.* Edinburgh, England: SHS Ltd.

Wagner, G.A. (1999). Further comments on person-centered approaches. *The Behavior Analyst, 22,* 53–54.

Wehmeyer, M.L. (1998). Self-determination and individuals with significant disabilities: Examining meanings and misinterpretations. *Journal of The Association for Persons with Severe Handicaps, 23,* 17–26.

References

Holburn, C.S. (2001). Compatibility of person-centered planning and applied behavior analysis. *The Behavior Analyst, 34,* 271–281.

Holburn, S., & Gordon, A. (2003). *Barriers to plan implementation form.* Staten Island: New York State Institute for Basic Research in Developmental Disabilities.

Holburn, S., Gordon, A., & Vietze, P. (2006). *Decision-making and satisfaction interview.* Staten Island: New York State Institute for Basic Research in Developmental Disabilities.

Holburn, C.S., Pfadt, A., Vietze, P., Schwartz, A.A., & Jacobson, J.W. (1996). *Person-centered planning quality of life indicators.* Staten Island: New York State Institute for Basic Research in Developmental Disabilities.

Holburn, C.S., Schwartz, A., & Jacobson, J.W. (1996). *Community activities checklist.* Albany, NY: Office of Mental Retardation and Developmental Disabilities.

Holburn, C.S., & Vietze, P. (1999). Acknowledging barriers in adopting person-centered planning. *Mental Retardation, 37,* 117–124.

Holburn, S., & Vietze, P. (2002). A better life for Hal: Five years of person-centered planning and applied behavior analysis with Hal. In S. Holburn & P.M. Vietze (Eds.), *Person-centered planning: Research, practice, and future directions* (pp. 291–314). Baltimore: Paul H. Brookes Publishing Co.

Holburn, C.S., Vietze, P., & Gordon, A. (2001). *Assessment of person-centered planning facilitation integrity.* Staten Island: New York State Institute for Basic Research in Developmental Disabilities.

Holburn, S., Vietze, P., Jacobson, J.W., & Gordon, A. (2003a). *Assessment of person-centered planning team integrity.* Staten Island: New York State Institute for Basic Research in Developmental Disabilities.

Holburn, S., Vietze, P., Jacobson, J.W., & Gordon, A. (2003b). *Person-centered organizational climate survey.* Staten Island: New York State Institute for Basic Research in Developmental Disabilities.

Kennedy, C.H., Horner, R.H., Newton, J.S., & Kanda, E. (1990). Measuring the activity patterns of adults with severe disabilities using the Resident Lifestyle Inventory. *The Journal of the Association for Persons with Severe Handicaps, 15,* 79–85.

Mount, B. (1992). *Person-centered planning: Finding directions for change. A sourcebook of values, ideals, and methods to encourage person-centered development.* New York: Graphic Futures.

Mount, B., & Patterson, J. (1986). *Update of the positive futures project: Initial outcomes and implications.* Hartford, CT: Department of Mental Retardation.

Nirje, B. (1969). The normalization principle and its human management implications. In R.B. Kugal & W. Wolfensberger (Eds.), *Changing patterns in residential services for the mentally retarded.* Washington, DC: President's Committee on Mental Retardation.

O'Brien, C.L., & O'Brien, J. (2002). The origins of person-centered planning: A community of practice perspective. In S. Holburn & P. Vietze (Eds.), *Person-centered planning: Research, practice, and future directions* (pp. 2–27). Baltimore: Paul H. Brookes Publishing Co.

O'Brien, J. (1987). A guide to life-style planning: Using the Activities Catalogue to integrate services and natural support systems. In G.T. Bellamy & B. Wilcox (Eds.), *A comprehensive guide to the Activities Catalogue: An alternative curriculum for youth and adults with severe disabilities* (pp. 175–189). Baltimore: Paul H. Brookes Publishing Co.

O'Brien, J., & Lovett, H. (1992). *Finding a way toward everyday lives: The contribution of person-centered planning.* Harrisburg: Pennsylvania Office of Mental Retardation. (Available from the Research and Training Center on Community Living, Center on Human Policy, Syracuse University)

O'Brien, J., O'Brien, C.L., & Mount, B. (1997). Person-centered planning has arrived or has it? *Mental Retardation, 35,* 480–488.

Pfadt, A., & Holburn, C.S. (1996). Community-based supports for people with challenging behaviors. *The Habilitative Mental Healthcare Newsletter, 15*(1), 8–11.

Reid, D.H., Everson, J.M., & Green, C.W. (1999). A systematic evaluation of preferences identified through person-centered planning for people with profound multiple disabilities. *Journal of Applied Behavior Analysis, 32,* 467–477.

Sanderson, H. (2002). A plan is not enough: Exploring the development of person-centered teams. In S. Holburn & P.M. Vietze (Eds.), *Person-centered planning: Research, practice, and future directions* (pp. 97–126). Baltimore: Paul H. Brookes Publishing Co.

Schwartz, A.A., Jacobson, J.W., & Holburn, C.S. (2000). Defining person-centeredness. *Education and Training in Mental Retardation and Developmental Disabilities, 35,* 235–249.

Smull, M.W. (1998). Revisiting choice. In J. O'Brien & C.L. O'Brien (Eds.), *A little book about person-centered planning* (pp. 37–49). Toronto: Inclusion Press.

Smull M.W., & Lakin, K.C. (2002). Public policy and person-centered planning. In S. Holburn & P.M. Vietze (Eds.), *Person-centered planning: Research, practice, and future directions* (pp. 379–397). Baltimore: Paul H. Brookes Publishing Co.

Wehmeyer, M.L. (1998). Self-determination and individuals with significant disabilities: Examining meanings and misinterpretations. *Journal of The Association for Persons with Severe Handicaps, 23,* 17–26.

Wolfensberger, W. (1972). *The principle of normalization in human services.* Toronto: National Institute on Mental Retardation.

Yates, J. (1980). *Program design sessions.* Carver, MA: Author. (Available from the author, 68 North Main Street, Carver, MA 02320)

Index

Page references to figures and tables are indicated by *f* and *t*, respectively.